Case Presentations
in Clinical Tuberculosis

Case Presentations in Clinical Tuberculosis

Peter D.O. Davies

MA, DM, FRCP

Consultant Chest Physician, The Cardiothoracic Centre, Liverpool NHS Trust, Liverpool, UK

AND

L. Peter Ormerod

BSc, MD, FRCP

Consultant Chest Physician, Blackburn Royal Infirmary, Blackburn, Hyndburn and Ribble Valley Health Care NHS Trust, Blackburn, UK

A member of the Hodder Headline Group
LONDON · SYDNEY · AUCKLAND
Co-published in the USA by
Oxford University Press Inc., New York

First published in Great Britain in 1999 by
Arnold, a member of the Hodder Headline Group,
338 Euston Road, London NW1 3BH

http://www.arnoldpublishers.com

Distributed in the United States of America by
Oxford University Press Inc.,
198 Madison Avenue, New York, NY10016
Oxford is a registered trademark of Oxford University Press

British Library Cataloguing in Publication Data
A catalogue record for this book is available from the British Library

Library of Congress Cataloging-in-Publication Data
A catalog record for this book is available from the Library of Congress

ISBN 0 340 74159 7 (pb)

1 2 3 4 5 6 7 8 9 10

Commissioning Editor: Joanna Koster
Project Editor: Sarah de Souza
Production Editor: Wendy Rooke
Production Controller: Priya Gohil

Typeset in 11/13 Goudy by Photoprint, Torquay, Devon
Printed in Suffolk by St Edmondsbury Press
Bound in Bristol by JW Arrowsmith Ltd

What do you think about this book? Or any other Arnold title?
Please send your comments to feedback.arnold@hodder.co.uk

Dedication

This book is dedicated to TB Alert, a new charity for resourcing tuberculosis research and service work in the developing world. All royalties from sales of this book will be donated to TB Alert.

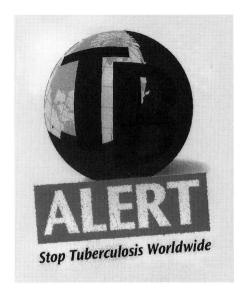

TB Alert
22 Tiverton Road
London
NW10 3HL
Tel: 0181 969 4830
Fax: 0181 960 0069
Email: tbalert@somhealy.demon.co.uk

Contents

About the authors

Peter Davies 'cut his teeth' on tuberculosis at the Medical Research Council's Tuberculosis and Chest Diseases Unit under Wallace Fox where he co-ordinated a survey of tuberculosis in the UK, and from which he wrote an MD thesis. Returning to clinical medicine, he continued to research aspects of the epidemiology of tuberculosis.

Soon after taking up a consultant appointment in Liverpool in 1988 he set up the Tuberculosis Research Unit in Liverpool. He is the editor of *Clinical Tuberculosis*, now in its second edition, and he co-authored the section on tuberculosis for the *Oxford Textbook of Medicine*, third edition. His interest in tuberculosis has led to extensive overseas lectures and visits, including acting for the World Health Organization in India.

Peter Ormerod had tuberculosis at the age of 7 years which made him decide to become a doctor. After qualifying in Manchester he underwent higher training there and in Birmingham. Since 1981 he has been Chest Physician in Blackburn, a high TB prevalence area of the UK, where he runs the tuberculosis service. In 1986 his MD thesis was on a personal series of 1000 tuberculosis cases. He has been a member of the Joint TB Committee of the British Thoracic Society since 1987 and is its current chairman. He is co-author of the UK national TB guidelines on treatment and on control and prevention, he advises a number of Government bodies, and he has published over 80 papers and articles on all aspects of tuberculosis, but with a particular focus on clinical, bacteriological and epidemiological aspects.

List of contributors

We would like to thank the following for contributing cases for inclusion.

Dr Nulda Beyers
University of Stellenbosch, Faculty of Medicine, PO Box 19063, 7505 Tyerberg, South Africa

Dr Sevetnana Bodi
Spitalul de Pediatrie 'St Maria', Str Bucium Nr 106, Iasi, Romania

Dr William J. Burman
Department of Public Health and Division of Infectious Diseases, University of Colorado Health Sciences Center, Denver, Colorado, USA

Dr Gary N. Carlos
De La Salle University Health Sciences Campus, Dasmarinas, Cavite, The Philippines

Professor Suchai Chareonratanakul
Division of Respiratory Disease and Tuberculosis, Faculty of Medicine, Siriraj Hospital, Bangkok 10700, Thailand

Dr Peter D.O. Davies
Tuberculosis Research Unit, Cardiothoracic Centre, Thomas Drive, Liverpool L14 3PE, UK

Professor D. Enarson
International Union Against Tuberculosis and Lung Disease (IUATLD), 68 Boulevard Saint-Michel, 75006 Paris, France

Dr Robert Gie
University of Stellenbosch, Faculty of Medicine, PO Box 19063, 7505 Tyerberg, South Africa

Dr N. Hargreaves
Department of Medicine, Lilongwe, Malawi

Professor A.D. Harries
c/o British High Commission, PO Box 30042, Lilongwe 3, Malawi

Dr Ashad Javaid
Department of Pulmonology, Postgraduate Medical Institute, Lady Reading Hospital, Peshawar, Pakistan

Dr Kittipong Maneechotesuwan
Division of Respiratory Disease and Tuberculosis, Faculty of Medicine, Siriraj Hospital, Bangkok 10700, Thailand

Dr L.P. Ormerod
Blackburn Royal Infirmary, Blackburn, UK
Dr Anton Pozniac
Department of Genito-Urinary Medicine, Chelsea and Westminster Hospital, 369 Fulham Road, Chelsea SW10 9NH, UK
Professor John A. Sbarbaro
Department of General Internal Medicine, University of Colorado Health Sciences Center, Denver, Colorado, USA
Dr Simon Schaaf
University of Stellenbosch, Faculty of Medicine, PO Box 19063, 7505 Tyerberg, South Africa
Dr C. Tam
Wanchai Polyclinic, Kennedy Road, Hong Kong
Dr Zarir Udwadia
Hinduja Hospital, Veer Savakar Marg, Bombay 400016, India
Dr Z. Wahbi
Aintree University Hospital, Long Lane, Liverpool, UK
Dr W.W. Yew
Tuberculosis and Chest Unit, Grantham Hospital, 125 Wong Chuk, Hang Road, Hong Kong
Dr Charles Yu
De La Salle University Health Sciences Campus, Dasmarinas, Cavite, The Philippines

Preface

Case presentations are probably the most enjoyable way to learn medicine. We have compiled this series of 120 cases in order to provide the reader with information about virtually every aspect of clinical tuberculosis.

The book covers the straightforward cases from initial diagnosis to discharge, the cases which are difficult to diagnose but easy to manage, problems of management in terms of poor compliance, adverse effects, emergent drug resistance and the development of concomitant disease. We have included some of our failures as well as our successes since, we reluctantly admit, we learn more from the former. Case management in some cases could have been improved upon, and where we believe this to be so, reference is made to better methods of management in the discussion. Where relevant we have included chest radiographs, histological findings and other clinical pictures. The reference sections are intended as a guide to further reading rather than as an exhaustive list of any relevant papers.

The emergence of HIV as the greatest risk factor for tuberculosis leading to disease has not only changed the epidemiology of tuberculosis beyond recognition, but has altered the clinical presentation as well. The section on HIV-positive disease is therefore relevant but represents only a small selection of the ways in which HIV-positive tuberculosis can present.

Cases are listed under the sections where they are likely to be most instructive. For example, a case of sputum-smear-positive pulmonary disease with hepatic failure will be listed under Risk Factors (hepatic failure) but cross-referenced to the relevant disease type (pulmonary sputum smear positive).

The book is intended to have an international flavour, so cases from many different countries are included. We are most grateful to all those who have provided cases. Wherever possible the consent of patients has been obtained before publishing medical details of their cases.

In the context of the world problem of tuberculosis this book is necessarily artificial. It is a type of 'detective book' in which most of the cases are difficult to diagnose. In contrast, the vast majority of tuberculosis world-wide occurs in smear-positive patients who are relatively easy to diagnose, provided that suitable microscopy services are available. The problem is not with the diagnosis, but with keeping the patient on treatment until he or she is cured.

Because this is a book of relative mysteries in tuberculosis, the X-ray, particularly the chest X-ray, is given prominence. However, in the context of the world burden of tuberculosis the X-ray may be an expensive luxury. It is the sputum smear which is the mainstay of diagnosis.

P.D.O. Davies
L.P. Ormerod
1999

Pulmonary disease

Case I The non-resolving pneumonia

Presenting complaint
A 25-year-old Pakistani man was admitted with 10 days of fever and cough but no sputum.

History of presenting complaint
The patient had previously been well and had not responded clinically to 5-day courses of erythromycin and cotrimoxazole prescribed by his family doctor. He had had fever for 10 days with a non-productive cough. He was a non-smoker.

Past medical history
He had no serious illness of note. His brother-in-law had had non-pulmonary tuberculosis 3 years previously.

Examination
He was febrile to 39.5°C and had signs of consolidation in the right upper zone and right mid zone. He weighed 64.9 kg.

Tests
His chest X-ray showed pneumonic shadowing in the right mid and upper zones without cavitation (Fig. 1.1). Serology for Legionnaires' disease and atypical pneumonias was negative. Erythrocyte sedimentation rate (ESR) was elevated at 86 mm/h.

Progress
The patient was treated with intravenous benzylpenicillin, a cephalosporin and erythromycin for 6 days without response. Bronchoscopy was then performed

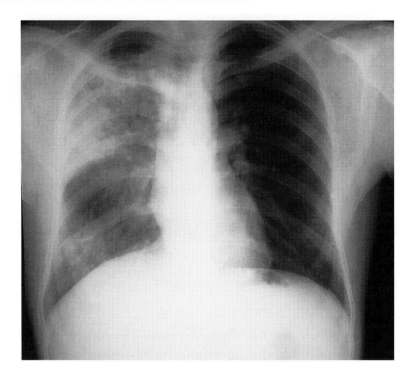

Fig. 1.1

which showed no endobronchial lesion, but washings were 3+ positive for acid-fast bacilli (AFB) on microscopy. Triple therapy with rifampicin/isoniazid and pyrazinamide was commenced, but he remained febrile over the next 10 days or so. Prednisolone 30 mg/day was added and the fever settled over the next 5 days. Steroids were gradually withdrawn, cultures were positive after 3 weeks, and full sensitivity was confirmed. Pyrazinamide was stopped after 2 months, and rifampicin/isoniazid were given for a further 4 months. At the end of treatment there was only minor X-ray scarring in the right upper zone, and the patient's weight was 78.8 kg.

Comment

Acute tuberculosis can present as simulating a bacterial pneumonia with a short history. Tuberculosis should be considered as a cause of non-resolving pneumonia. Bronchoscopy with washings for alveolar lavage are now well-accepted techniques for the investigation of suspected tuberculosis in individuals who cannot produce sputum. They also have the added advantage of excluding endobronchial disease and copathology, such as bronchial carcinoma in older smokers or ex-smokers. Those who are unable to produce sputum spontaneously, even though smear positive from washings, are of lower infectivity than those who are smear positive on spontaneously produced secretions. Such cases should be equated with smear-negative, culture-positive cases for the purposes of contact tracing.

References
Chawla, R., Pant, K., Jaggi, O.P. *et al.* 1988: Fibreoptic bronchoscopy in smear-negative pulmonary tuberculosis. *European Respiratory Journal* 1, 804–6.

Willcox, P.A., Benatar, S.R., Potgeiter, P.D. 1982: Use of the flexible fibreoptic bronchoscope in the diagnosis of sputum-negative pulmonary tuberculosis. *Thorax* 37, 598–601.

Case 2 The lady with the weak and painful voice

Presenting complaint
A 52-year-old white woman presented with a weak and painful voice.

History of presenting complaint
The patient had had asthma for over 20 years and was on treatment with regular inhaled beclomethasone 400 μg bd. For the previous 8 weeks she had a cough productive of a cupful of sputum daily, and she had developed a painful and weak voice. An ear, nose and throat (ENT) examination shortly after the onset of symptoms showed no laryngeal lesion. There was no history of previous cough or sputum production, and the patient was a non-smoker. Forced expiratory volume in 1 s (FEV_1) was 1.7/2.4 L.

Tests
Chest X-ray (Fig. 2.1) showed minimal shadowing in the right middle lobe, raising the possibility of bronchiectasis. Tests for allergic bronchopulmonary aspergillosis were negative, with no radio-allergosorbant (RAST)-specific IgE to aspergillus and no blood eosinophilia. The patient's weight was 41.6 kg.

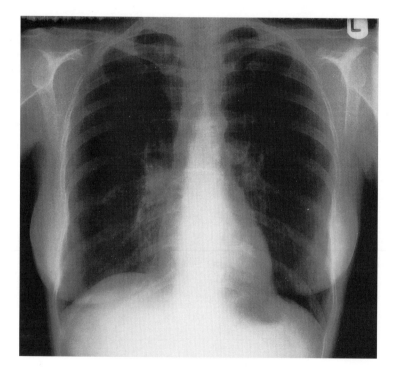

Fig. 2.1

Progress

It was thought unlikely that the patient's weak voice was related to the inhaled corticosteroids, as she had been taking these for several years and her larynx was also painful. Although the X-ray showed little shadowing and no cavitation, sputum was examined for AFB and was found to be 3+ positive. Triple therapy was commenced and liver function was normal. After 3 weeks, nausea developed and biochemical hepatitis was shown (bilirubin 32 mg/L; alanine aminotransferase (ALT) 3160 IU/L). Rifampicin, isoniazid and pyrazinamide were stopped and ethambutol 15 mg/kg and streptomycin 0.5 g daily were given until the patient's liver function returned to normal. Isoniazid was reintroduced at 50 mg/day for 3 days, and then at 300 mg daily without problems. Rifampicin was then reintroduced at 150 mg daily for 3 days and then at 450 mg daily with liver function remaining normal. Streptomycin was then stopped, but hepatitis again developed (ALT 1210 IU/L). Rifampicin and isoniazid were again stopped until liver function returned to normal with ethambutol and streptomycin cover. Isoniazid was reintroduced in increasing dosages without further hepatitis. Cultures confirmed full sensitivity. The hepatitis was thought to be most probably due to rifampicin. Treatment was continued with isoniazid and ethambutol for a further 7 months. Cultures were negative after 6 months of treatment, and again 6 months after stopping treatment.

Comment

Tuberculous laryngitis is usually painful and responds rapidly to antituberculosis drugs. It is usually found complicating extensive smear-positive pulmonary disease. Occasionally it can be found with smear-positive disease without cavitation, when it is presumed to be an endobronchial focus, in this case thought to be at the middle lobe junction, and ruptures into the bronchial tree discharging tuberculous material directly into the bronchus. This case was further complicated by the development of drug-related hepatitis. Because of smear-positive disease (i.e. an infectious case), treatment with non-hepatotoxic antituberculosis drugs was given until liver function returned to normal. As full sensitivity had been demonstrated, treatment with isoniazid/ethambutol was used for the continuation phase, but with close supervision.

Reference

Ip, M.S.M., Yo, S.Y. and Lam, W.K. et al. 1986: Endobronchial tuberculosis revisited. *Chest* **89**, 727–30.

Cross reference

Chapter 2, Management of adverse drug reactions

Case 3   The home carer

Presenting complaint
A 35-year-old female East European immigrant presented with 2 months of cough and malaise.

History of presenting complaint
The patient, a nurse, had emigrated from Eastern Europe to the UK 5 years previously. She worked as a carer in a local residential home for the elderly and lived with her husband and two children, aged 4 and 6 years. Two months before presentation she began to feel unwell and developed a persistent irritating cough. She lost approximately 5 kg in weight. She also experienced night sweats and low-grade pyrexia. There was no significant past history.

Examination
The patient appeared well and had no abnormal physical findings.

Tests
A chest X-ray, performed at the request of the general practitioner, showed a 5-cm cavitating lesion at the left apex (Figs 3.1 and 3.2). The radiographer

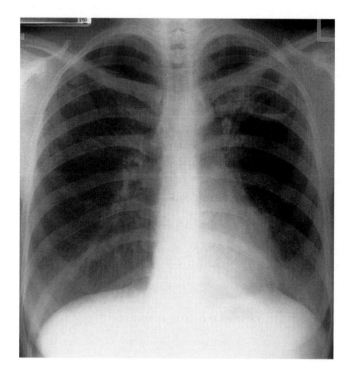

Fig. 3.1

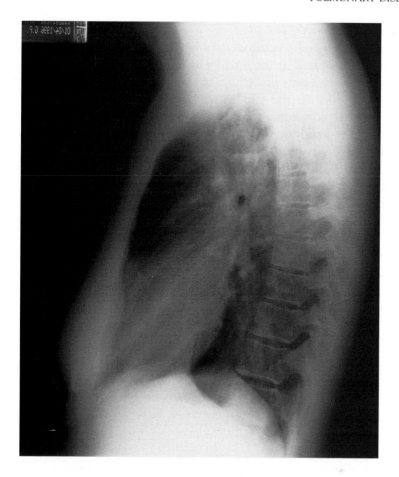

Fig. 3.2

showed the film to the duty radiologist, who immediately telephoned the local physician with an interest in tuberculosis. The patient was seen in the clinic that afternoon. She was sent home with three sputum pots. On her return with the pots 3 days later the tuberculin test performed in the clinic showed a 20-mm induration to 10 IU. The patient started treatment on Rifater and ethambutol. All three pots were strongly positive on direct smear and grew *Mycobacterium tuberculosis*, fully sensitive to all first-line drugs.

Outcome

The patient made an uneventful recovery. Therapy was reduced to isoniazid and rifampicin when culture results became available, and stopped after 6 months. On contact tracing the patient's children were found to be tuberculin test positive but clear of active disease, and were given 3 months of preventive therapy (isoniazid and rifampicin). Tracing at the residential home where the patient worked revealed no further cases.

Comment

Fortunately the general practitioner strongly suspected tuberculosis and a chest radiograph was obtained at the first opportunity. An alert radiographer was able to activate the appropriate procedures so that the patient was seen by a specialist as soon as possible. As the patient was reasonably well, and able to produce sputum, hospital admission for medical and nursing care or diagnosis was unnecessary. Her family would already have been infected, so isolation at this stage would have served no useful purpose, although she was told not to go to work, leave the house or meet anyone new, especially children, until her treatment had started. The level of clinical suspicion was high enough for the consultant physician to start her on treatment as soon as specimens for microbiology had been obtained. In fact, confirmation of the diagnosis was obtained an hour or so later.

The patient had worked as a hospital nurse in her native country, and therefore had two social risk factors for disease, namely country of origin and occupation. As the infection had probably been acquired abroad, where drug resistance is common, she was started on four drugs.

Case 4   The persistent tramp

Presenting complaint
A 56-year-old homeless man was admitted in a confused and semi-comatose state via the casualty department. Little history was available, but he had apparently been 'living rough' on the city streets for some time when he was found and picked up by the ambulance crew.

Examination
Physical examination showed a dishevelled and cachexic man who had obviously been living rough for some time. His weight was 38 kg. He was pyrexial with a temperature of 39°C. His pulse rate was 110 beats/min, and blood pressure (BP) was 90/0 mmHg. There were diminished breath sounds throughout the left lung, with an area of bronchial breathing at the apex. There were numerous superficial sores on the patient's arms and legs.

Tests
A chest X-ray showed extensive shadowing throughout the left lung, and patchy shadowing in the upper third of the right lung, with at least one large (5-cm) cavity (Fig. 4.1). The patient's sputum was teeming with acid- and alcohol-fast bacilli (AAFB) on direct smear.

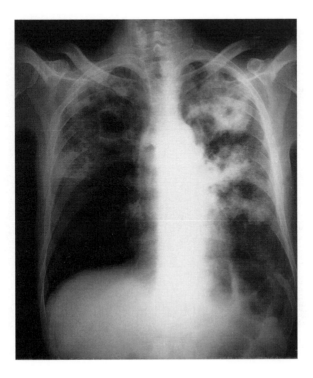

Fig. 4.1

Progress

The patient was started on triple therapy, isoniazid, rifampicin and pyrazinamide. The initial clinical course was stormy. His blood pressure fell to 60/0 mmHg. A short synacthen test was normal, but the patient was commenced on high-dose oral prednisolone, 40 mg/day. He developed a deep-vein thrombosis in his right leg, for which he was treated with warfarin for 6 weeks. He was very reluctant to eat at first, and special diets had to be requested. During 3 months of intensive in-patient treatment he gradually improved and was able to care for himself. Despite adequate therapy for a fully susceptible organism and satisfactory clinical response, his sputum remained smear positive for AAFB. However, by the end of the fourth month of therapy the cultures had reverted to negative. There was complete resolution of shadowing in the right lung, and contraction of the left lung, leaving a hilar scar (Fig. 4.2). The patient was therefore discharged to warden-controlled accommodation where arrangements were made for him to have directly observed therapy.

Treatment was continued for 9 months. Three months after completion of treatment the patient was readmitted because of general malaise. He had not lost any weight since discharge but sputum was again positive for AAFB. There had been no appreciable change in his chest X-ray since his discharge. Once again this remained culture negative at 12 weeks' incubation. He was discharged home on no treatment.

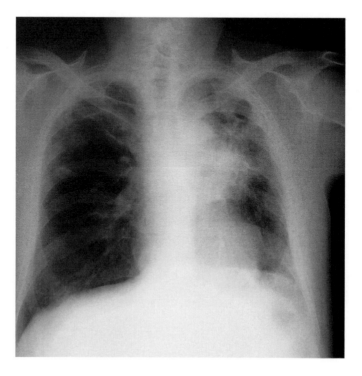

Fig. 4.2

Comment

This patient showed all the characteristics of the vagrant. He had extensive smear-positive disease and very nearly died within a short time of the treatment being started. He eventually responded well, but continues to cough up mycobacteria that the laboratory has been unable to culture. This is sometimes seen following cure of extensive radiographic disease, and is probably due to the large numbers of M. *tuberculosis* organisms which have been killed by treatment continuing to be eliminated for months afterwards. The problem is that direct smear cannot distinguish between live and dead organisms, and therefore the patient had to be treated as though he had active disease. Appropriate public-health measures, including contact tracing, had to be undertaken until it was certain that the organisms were not viable M. *tuberculosis*, and that the patient was non-infectious.

Alternatively, an environmental mycobacterium, which was not viable under the laboratory conditions used for culture, could have invaded the abscess cavities and scarring in the previously diseased lungs and caused the patient to expectorate AAFB that were indistinguishable from M. *tuberculosis* on direct smear. Environmental mycobacteria such as M. *xenopi* or M. *kansasii* commonly colonize a cavity caused by previous infection by M. *tuberculosis*, and may cause disease clinically similar to tuberculosis (see Chapter 10, p. 259).

Reference

Vidalm, R., Martin-Casabona, N., Juan, A., Falgueras, T. and Miravitlles, M. 1996: Incidence and significance of acid-fast bacilli in sputum smears at the end of antituberculous treatment. *Chest* **109**, 1562–5.

Case 5   Like grandfather, like grandson

Presenting complaint
The patient was diagnosed in the tuberculosis screening clinic after his grandson had been diagnosed as having tuberculosis.

History of presenting complaint
The patient, a 57-year-old white man, had had tuberculosis as a child. For 12 months prior to presentation his smoker's cough had become more persistent. He had been losing weight and felt generally unwell. He also complained of night sweats. On several occasions he had suggested tuberculosis to his family doctor but had been reassured on the grounds that 'nobody gets tuberculosis these days.' In the month before he presented he had developed a painful throat and hoarse voice.

His 8-year-old grandson had become progressively more unwell during the previous 3 months and was referred to hospital after a chest X-ray had shown right middle lobe collapse. A tuberculin test had been very strongly positive. At diagnosis his family contacts were quickly traced and his immediate family was seen at the contact clinic within a few days. It was at this time that the grandfather's diagnosis was made.

Tests
A chest X-ray performed in the clinic showed extensive left upper lobe disease with a 4-cm cavity (Fig. 5.1). Subsequent sputum specimens were heavily stained with AAFB which cultured positive as M. *tuberculosis*.

Outcome
The patient was advised to come into hospital for the start of treatment, as it was felt that the extent of disease was such that medical complications could arise. He refused to be hospitalized, and started triple therapy (isoniazid, rifampicin and pyrazinamide) as an out-patient. One week later he suffered a severe haemoptysis and was admitted as an emergency, but the bleeding stopped and he was discharged after 2 weeks. During follow-up he was also diagnosed as having asthma and bird-fancier's lung, for which high-dose oral steroids (60 mg/day) were given for 2 months. Following discharge the patient made a generally uncomplicated recovery from the tuberculosis.

Comment
This patient was diagnosed at the screening clinic after his grandson had presented with disease. From the length of the case histories and contact history there is little doubt that the grandfather had infected the child. Restriction fragment length polymorphism (RFLP) testing was not routinely available in the area to confirm this at the time.

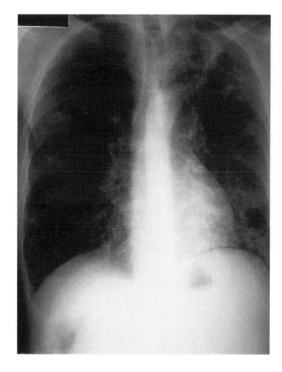

Fig. 5.1

In the city in which these patients resided, 50 per cent of children with tuberculosis are found as a result of screening close contacts of an adult with disease. In this case the index case, namely the grandfather, was found after the child had first presented. This is unusual, but occurred because the patient's medical practitioner had not considered the possibility of tuberculosis.

The case illustrates the importance of contact tracing children, not because they are likely to have infected anyone, but because they can be evidence of an undetected index case.

Tuberculosis in children aged 6–14 years is usually a relatively benign disease and often asymptomatic, but potentially fatal tuberculous meningitis may occur at this age, particularly in the UK, where BCG vaccination is not routinely given until the age of 12–13 years.

Cross reference
Chapter 7, Childhood disease

Case 6 Three cases: three generations

Presenting complaint
A 68-year-old man, his 43-year-old son and 18-month-old grandson all presented with tuberculosis on the same day.

History of presenting complaint
The grandfather had had pulmonary tuberculosis 13 years previously. For 3 months up until presentation he had complained of cough, weight loss and malaise with night sweats. His son, an unemployed labourer, had had a very similar history with 2 months of cough, weight loss and malaise. Both had presented to their general practitioner on the same day. They had been sent for a chest X-ray to their nearest hospital, where the X-ray department had contacted the admitting medical team (Figs 6.1 and 6.2). Both men were admitted and sputum sent off in casualty was reported to be smear positive for AAFB. As a result, the general practitioner also sent the grandson, who was asymptomatic, to the children's hospital to be screened. A chest X-ray showed right middle lobe collapse (Fig. 6.3) and a tuberculin test was very strongly positive.

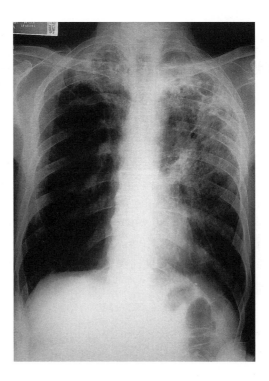

Fig. 6.1

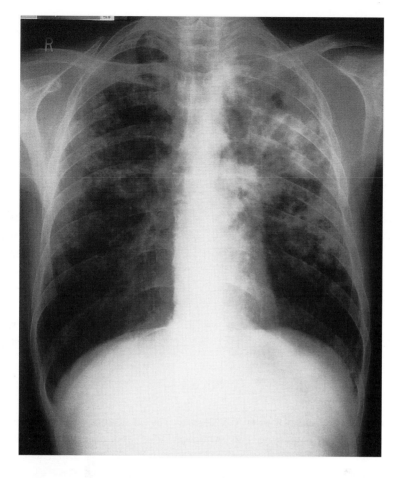

Fig. 6.2

Outcome

All three patients made a satisfactory recovery on 6 months of standard chemotherapy. The isolates were fully sensitive to all first-line drugs. Screening of the rest of the household showed that the wife of the grandfather also had pulmonary disease. She was asymptomatic, with only a small area of consolidation in the left lung. Only the wife of the son (i.e. the mother of the grandson) was free of disease, but in view of the extent of disease in the family and the fact that she had a grade-4 Heaf test, she was given 3 months of preventive therapy consisting of isoniazid and rifampicin.

Comment

This is a clear example of the way in which tuberculosis can spread within a household if it is not considered by either the patient or his or her general practitioner. In this case the grandfather had had disease previously but failed to present to the medical services due to fear of possible lung cancer (he was also

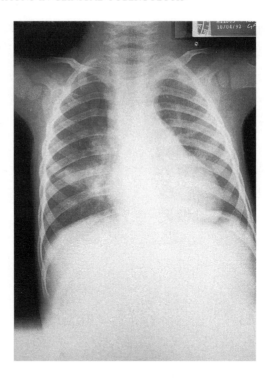

Fig. 6.3

a heavy smoker). It was not until the disease was far advanced in both men that they presented. By this time the grandson also had extensive disease. Fortunately, this was contained as primary pulmonary disease and the child was well. Tuberculosis at this age (18 months) may well disseminate to the brain, meninges or other parts of the body with potentially (and rapidly) fatal consequences.

Approximately 10 per cent of tuberculosis in the UK occurs in people with previously treated disease. At least half of these will have been treated for a previous infection abroad, and have probably relapsed rather than acquired a new infection. The proportion of native English people who relapse is unclear, but is probably about 5 per cent. Although there are no firm data, it is suggested that those treated with a non-rifampicin-containing regimen are more likely to relapse than those who had received rifampicin as part of their initial regimen. Tuberculosis is more likely to occur in those who have had previous disease. This may be attributed to patients not taking their medication as prescribed. Trials of the most effective regimes still show a 1 to 2 per cent relapse rate.

References
Chan, S.L. and Yew, W.W. 1998: Chemotherapy. In Davies, P.D.O. (ed.), *Chemotherapy in clinical tuberculosis*, 2nd edn. London: Chapman and Hall, 243–64.

Kumar, D., Watson, J.M., Charlett, A., Nicholas, S. and Darbyshire, J.H. 1997: Tuberculosis in England and Wales; results of a national survey. *Thorax* **52**, 1060–7.

Cross reference
Chapter 7, Childhood disease

Case 7   The Chinese local

Presenting complaint
A 16-year-old Chinese girl presented with a 2-year history of painful swelling on the shins.

History of presenting complaint
The patient had been born to Chinese parents in the UK and, apart from two visits to Hong Kong at the age of 10 and 14 years, had lived in the UK all her life. At the age of 14 years she noticed painful swelling on both shins (erythema nodosum, Plate 7.1), and was referred by her general practitioner to a hospital specialist. After extensive investigation no clear cause of the erythema nodosum was found, and the patient was eventually referred to a chest physician for investigation of a possible diagnosis of tuberculosis. At presentation she was entirely asymptomatic apart from evident erythema nodosum confined to both shins. The patient had had BCG vaccination at birth. On routine school testing at the age of 12 years the tuberculin test was weakly positive, so further BCG vaccination was not given.

Tests
A chest X-ray showed minimal lung shadowing around the left hilum. A tuberculin test was strongly positive. A bronchoscopy was normal, but washings were positive for AAFB on direct smear. These subsequently grew M. *tuberculosis* that was sensitive to all first-line drugs.

Outcome
The patient was started on standard triple therapy after the bronchoscopy. There was resolution of the X-ray shadowing and regression of the erythema nodosum. The patient was left with some permanent discoloration of the shins.

Comment
Tuberculosis is a well-known cause of erythema nodosum. In the case of this patient it was not considered for a long time because the attending doctors may have been misled by the patient's strong regional English accent. Children born to ethnic minority groups in the UK are at increased risk of tuberculosis, although not to the same extent as those born in their country of origin. The reason is probably because of visits back to the country of origin, as was almost certainly the case with this patient. Other important causes of erythema nodosum are infections, particularly due to *Streptococcus*, and sarcoidosis.

Erythema nodosum is associated with primary tuberculosis, and usually develops within 6 weeks of the initial infection, at about the same time as the tuberculin skin test becomes positive. It is thought to be due to a hypersensitivity phenomenon, as bacilli are not found in the lesions. Following UK guidelines this patient was given BCG vaccination at birth, which is recommended for children born to groups at increased risk of tuberculosis. Protection afforded by BCG vaccination is only about 75 per cent at best, and lasts for only 15 years. Although the patient may have benefited from a second vaccination at the age of 12 years (when it is routinely given to children in the UK with no specific risk factors for tuberculosis), there is no evidence to suggest that protection is conferred by second or subsequent vaccinations. The weakly positive tuberculin test that this patient had 2 years before she presumably acquired the infection is no guide to the protective effect of vaccination.

References

Salisbury, D.M. and Begg, N.T. eds. 1996: Tuberculosis: BCG immunisation. In *Immunisation against infectious disease*. London, Cardiff, Edinburgh and Belfast: Department of Health, Welsh Office, Scottish Office DOH and DHSS (Northern Ireland), 219–41.

Smith, P.G. and Fine, P.E.M. 1998: BCG vaccination. In Davies, P.D.O. (ed.), *Clinical tuberculosis*, 2nd edn. Chapman and Hall, London, 417–34.

Case 8 The tuberculous 'tongue'

Presenting complaint
A 43-year-old woman presented with worsening cough and persistent weight loss.

History of presenting complaint
The patient, who had smoked 40 cigarettes a day for more than 20 years, noticed that her smoker's cough was becoming more persistent and troublesome. She also felt progressively more unwell and had lost a few kilograms in weight. She had had no significant history of previous disease, but thought that her father might have died of tuberculosis when she was in her early teens. Physical examination was unremarkable.

Tests
Postero-anterior and lateral chest X-rays showed extensive shadowing confined to the lingular lobe (lingua = tongue in Latin) (Figs 8.1 and 8.2). Sputum was positive for AAFB on direct smear, so a bronchoscopy, which had been requested to exclude a lung tumour, was cancelled and the patient was started on triple therapy.

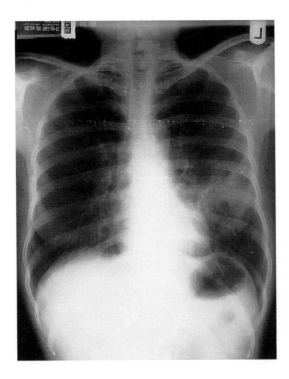

Fig. 8.1

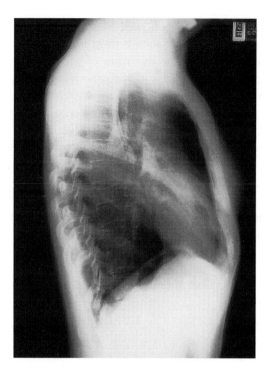

Fig. 8.2

Progress
Although she continued to take the drug regimen as prescribed (isoniazid, rifampicin and pyrazinamide for 2 months, followed by isoniazid and rifampicin for 4 months), she continued to experience several symptoms during treatment, including continuing malaise, cough, nausea, weakness and chest pains. Three months into therapy she was admitted to hospital with severe sudden left-sided chest pains. A bronchoscopy and ventilation perfusion lung scan performed at this time were normal. The patient became smear and culture negative after 3 months of therapy.

Her physical well-being improved slightly after the end of therapy. Lingular shadowing persisted after the end of therapy, but has continued to improve on follow-up. She continued to smoke at least 40 cigarettes a day throughout treatment, despite repeated advice to stop smoking.

Comment
Post-primary tuberculosis, the form that is usually seen in adults, tends to be posterior apical in distribution. Why this is so is unclear, but it may be linked to the area of the lung with maximal aeration and minimal perfusion. If a single lobe segment is affected, the commonest segments are the posterior segment of the upper lobe and the apical segment. The next commonest is probably the

apical segment of the lower lobe, followed by the anterior upper lobe segment. Shadowing confined to the lingular lobe is most unusual, so lung carcinoma was by far the most likely diagnosis at the time of presentation. Fortunately, the resident who first saw the patient was alert to the possibility of tuberculosis, and sent off sputum for the appropriate tests.

Because of her persistent chest pains, heavy smoking and unusual site of infection, a bronchoscopy and computerized tomography (CT) scan were performed after 3 months, but no evidence of tumour was found. The cause of the chest pains was never established, but was presumed to be musculoskeletal in nature, and brought on by coughing.

The possibility of dual-disease tuberculosis and lung cancer should always be borne in mind. There may be an increased risk of cancer formation in the scar caused by tuberculosis of the lung.

Reference

Simon, G. 1962: *Principles of chest X-ray diagnosis*, 2nd edn. London: Butterworths.

Case 9   A Chinese puzzle: double diagnosis

Presenting complaint
A 64-year-old Chinese man presented with cough and haemoptysis.

History of presenting complaint
The patient had emigrated from Hong Kong to the UK 30 years previously. He had been generally fit in the past, but 3 months before presentation he developed a persistent cough. Latterly there had been flecks of blood mixed in the sputum. He had also lost about 7 kg in weight. He was a heavy smoker, and had smoked about 30 cigarettes a day for all of his adult life.

Tests
A chest X-ray showed a cavitating lesion in the right upper lobe (Fig. 9.1). The patient was unable to produce sputum, so a fibrotic bronchoscopy was performed. No abnormality was found, but washings were positive on direct smear for AAFB. There was no sign of malignant cells in the washings.

Progress
The patient was started on quadruple therapy for tuberculosis, consisting of isoniazid, rifampicin, pyrazinamide and ethambutol. He initially made good

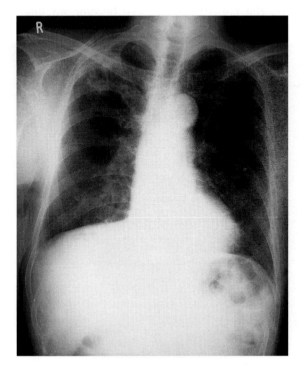

Fig. 9.1

progress, but 6 weeks after treatment had started he was admitted to hospital with a fracture of the right humerus (Fig. 9.2). A biopsy showed squamous-cell carcinoma, presumably of bronchogenic origin. The patient was treated with radiotherapy to the arm and lesion in the right upper lobe, which had not changed during the period of treatment. He eventually died 4 months later of disseminated carcinoma. His antituberculous chemotherapy was continued throughout.

Comment

This patient suffered from carcinoma of the lung and tuberculosis simultaneously. In societies where smoking is common, this is not an infrequent occurrence. Squamous-cell carcinoma frequently presents with a cavitating lesion. The finding of AAFB at bronchoscopy naturally led to a diagnosis of tuberculosis, and a second diagnosis of carcinoma was not considered until the patient presented with a pathological fracture of the humerus. Although tuberculosis of the long bones does occur, the development of a fracture 6 weeks into treatment raised suspicion of a carcinoma, which was confirmed on bone biopsy. The only treatment available at this stage was palliation. Radiotherapy was given to reduce tumour size, but healing of the humerus did not take place before death. The patient received continued treatment for tuberculosis because if that treatment had been withdrawn the spread of tuberculosis might have been rapid. Furthermore, the patient would have become an infectious risk to his

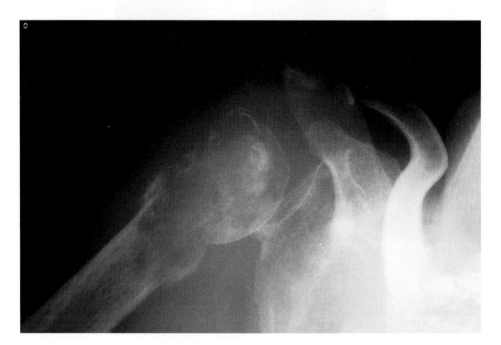

Fig. 9.2

immediate family. The coincidence of two pathologies is always confusing. It is likely that the development of lung cancer occurred first and lowered the patient's immunity, resulting in a recrudescence of old tuberculosis infection acquired earlier in Hong Kong.

There is an approximately threefold increased risk of tuberculosis in smokers.

References

Tocque, K., Remmington, T., Beeching, N.J. *et al.* 1997: Case-control study of lifestyle risk factors for tuberculosis in Liverpool, UK. *Thorax* **52** (Suppl. 6), A34.

Yu, G., Hsieh, C. and Peng, J. 1988: Risk factors associated with the prevalence of pulmonary tuberculosis among sanitary workers in Shanghai. *Tubercle* **69**, 105–12.

Cross reference
Chapter 11, Altered diagnosis

Case 10   The late relapse

Presenting complaint
A 71-year-old woman presented with cough, malaise and weight loss.

History of presenting complaint
The patient had had tuberculosis as a young adult and remembered receiving a long course of injections and drinks containing medication. She had been a life-long smoker, and in the previous few years had had recurrent bouts of acute or chronic bronchitis. She was on a number of medications, including an inhaler containing a steroid. She had been having regular follow-up in the clinic for her chronic bronchitis, and prior to her current presentation had had an appointment 1 year previously. At presentation she complained of 3 months of an increasingly harsh cough which had not responded to several courses of antibiotics prescribed by her general practitioner. She had become progressively more unwell and had begun to lose weight (about 3 kg) between clinic visits.

Tests
The patient's chest X-rays taken before presentation had consistently shown bilateral upper zone spotted calcification as a result of her earlier tuberculosis. This had remained stable for many years (Fig. 10.1). The new chest X-ray taken

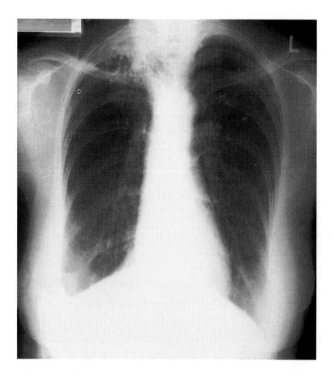

Fig. 10.1

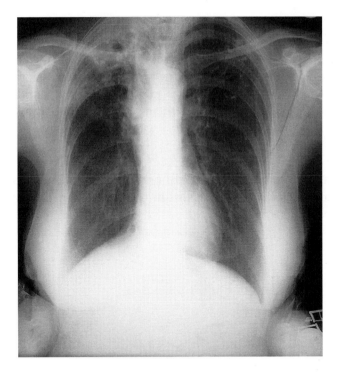

Fig. 10.2

at current presentation with new symptoms clearly showed fresh cavitation at the right apex (Fig. 10.2). The sputum was positive for AAFB.

Outcome

The patient was started on triple therapy consisting of isoniazid, rifampicin and pyrazinamide, and she made an uneventful recovery. Treatment was reduced to isoniazid and rifampicin after 2 months and was stopped after 6 months.

Comment

Approximately 10 per cent of patients treated for tuberculosis in the UK have received treatment for a previous episode of disease. It has been assumed that these are patients who have had a non-rifampicin-containing regimen previously, but there is no good evidence for this. Current guidelines recommend a four-drug regimen for cases of relapse, in case there is resistance to one or two drugs in the new regimen. Drug resistance among white relapse patients in the UK is very rare, and is usually to streptomycin alone. From this patient's history she almost certainly had been given streptomycin and para-aminosalicylic acid (PAS) at her initial treatment, and would therefore be in no danger of having an organism resistant to the newer drugs being used to treat this episode.

There is much controversy as to whether steroids precipitate a relapse of tuberculosis by reducing the host immunity to M. *tuberculosis*. There is anecdotal evidence but no good statistical evidence that this is the case. The steroid inhaler was providing a daily dose of only 400 µg prednisolone daily. We do not normally recommend prophylaxis for patients with a history of tuberculosis and radiographic evidence of healed disease who are about to start a course of steroids. However, where a high dose is prescribed over a period of time, e.g. 1 mg/kg for over 1 month, special care should be taken to follow up the patient closely.

Reference

Joint Tuberculosis Committee of the British Thoracic Society. 1998: Chemotherapy and management of tuberculosis in the United Kingdom: recommendations. *Thorax* **53**, 536–48.

SECTION IB SMEAR-NEGATIVE, CULTURE-POSITIVE DISEASE

Case 11 I haven't got over the flu, doctor

Presenting complaint
A 66-year-old white woman presented with malaise after a 'flu-like' illness.

History of presenting complaint
Three months previously the patient had had a flu-like illness with myalgia, mild fever and malaise. She had had a productive cough for about 1 week but this had settled, she had lost only 1.5 kg in weight, and she had no fever or sweats but just felt 'below par'. She smoked 10 cigarettes a day.

Past medical history
The patient had had pneumonia 8 years previously, but had been told that the X-ray had largely cleared. She had had a hip replacement 3 years earlier. An aunt had died of tuberculosis when the patient was aged 8 years, 58 years previously.

Tests
Chest X-ray showed some infiltration in the right upper zone, but there was also some loss of volume and scarring, with the trachea slightly deviated to the right (Fig. 11.1). Haemoglobin was 12.6 g/dL, ESR was 30 mm/h and globulin was raised at 41 g/L. There was no sputum to test.

Progress
A fibre-optic bronchoscopy was performed in order to exclude proximal bronchial carcinoma and to obtain washings from the right upper lobe. No endobronchial lesion was seen. Washings from the right upper lobe bronchus were negative on microscopy for AFB. The patient was observed initially, but after 4 weeks washings were culture-positive for M. tuberculosis, later confirmed as fully sensitive to all first-line drugs. Treatment was commenced with triple therapy (isoniazid, rifampicin and pyrazinamide). Some itching occurred, but no rash, which was controlled by concurrent antihistamine administration. Liver function was normal. Standard short-course chemotherapy was given for 6 months. The X-ray showed some resolution, but some scarring remained.

Comment
This was almost certainly reactivation disease following earlier infection. The symptoms of early disease can be non-specific. The chest X-ray shows the extent of the area involved by disease or scarring, but the activity of disease is judged from respiratory secretions and not from an X-ray report. Bronchoscopy excluded coexistent bronchial carcinoma but gave the diagnosis. Washings for AFB

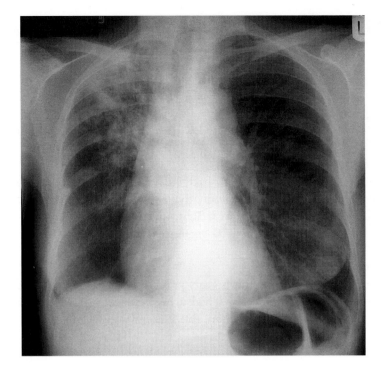

Fig. 11.1

culture should be taken routinely from upper lobe lesions without endobronchial disease, as these show unsuspected tuberculosis in a number of cases.

Mild itching without rash occurs in a small percentage of cases, and is normally attributable to the pyrazinamide. This can usually be managed by symptomatic treatment with antihistamines, and the patient should be advised that if pyrazinamide has to be withdrawn, treatment will have to be extended from 6 to 9 months.

Reference
Ip, M., Chau, P.Y., So, S.Y. *et al.* 1989: The value of routine bronchial aspirate culture at fibreoptic bronchoscopy for the diagnosis of tuberculosis. *Tubercle* **79**, 281–5.

Cross reference
Chapter 2, Management of adverse drug reactions

Case 12   Don't just go on the X-ray

Presenting complaint
An 83-year-old white man was seen with streak haemoptysis and a weight loss of 5 kg.

History of presenting complaint
The patient had had mucoid sputum with streak haemoptysis for 2 months, during which time he had also felt rather unwell with loss of appetite and he had lost 5 kg. He had not experienced chest pain or any increase in breathlessness. He was a non-smoker with no previous medical history, and he had never attended a hospital or had a chest X-ray before.

Examination
The patient weighed 76 kg, and there were no focal signs in the chest and no other findings on general examination.

Tests
His chest X-ray showed multiple calcified areas in both lungs and in both upper and lower zones (Fig. 12.1), and had been reported as 'old tuberculous calcified

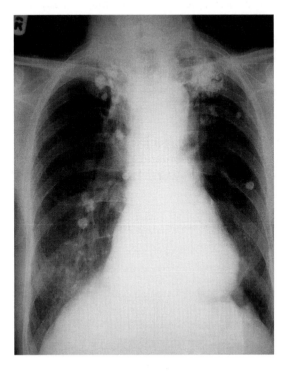

Fig. 12.1

foci; no evidence of activity'. Haemoglobin was 11.8 g/dL normochromic with an ESR of 36 mm/h. Biochemistry was normal.

Progress
Three sputum samples were collected, but all were negative on microscopy for AFB. The patient was observed for 4 weeks when his chest X-ray had not changed. Sputum was culture positive at 4 weeks for M. *tuberculosis*. Treatment with rifampicin, isoniazid and pyrazinamide was commenced pending sensitivity results. These drugs were given for 2 months, by which time full sensitivity was confirmed. Pyrazinamide was then stopped, and rifampicin/isoniazid were continued for a further 4 months. The patient rapidly recovered his appetite and regained weight. His chest X-ray at the end of treatment was identical to that at the beginning of treatment and to all subsequent X-rays.

Comment
Despite the chest X-ray report, the patient's family practitioner was not satisfied that things really were inactive. The chest X-ray indicates the *extent* of the problem, but does not reliably define *activity*. The definition of inactivity is three negative sputum cultures *and* failure of any chest X-ray features to worsen over time. In developed countries tuberculosis is often a disease of the elderly in the white ethnic group, representing reactivation of disease acquired earlier in life. If such calcified lesions as were present on this man's X-ray are removed at post-mortem and injected into guinea-pigs, viable tubercle bacilli can be recovered from a small percentage of animals. This provides the rationale for chemoprophylaxis with isoniazid in asymptomatic cases, with 6- or 12-month regimens having been shown to be effective (International Union Against Tuberculosis Committee on Prophylaxis, 1982).

Reference
International Union Against Tuberculosis Committee on Prophylaxis. 1982: Efficacy of various durations of isoniazid preventive therapy for tuberculosis: 5 years of follow-up. *Bulletin of the World Health Organization* **60**, 555–64.

Case 13 Lumps on the legs

Presenting complaint
A 33-year-old women of mixed race was referred with erythema nodosum that had been present for 6 weeks.

History of presenting complaint
The patient was born in the UK of Afro-Caribbean and white parents and worked in the nursing profession. About 6 weeks earlier she had noticed bruise-like swellings on the anterior shins which had 'come and gone' since that time. She denied weight loss, cough or iritis. She had had a BCG vaccination at the age of 13 years and had had an appropriate tuberculin test at the start of her nursing training. She was currently working in a nursing home for the elderly. The patient had no previous medical history.

Examination
There was definite erythema nodosum present on both shins, but none on the thighs or forearms. There was no peripheral lymphadenopathy, iritis, parotid enlargement or hepatosplenomegaly. There were no focal signs in the lungs.

Tests
Haemoglobin was 13.2 g/dL normochromic and ESR was 54 mm/h. Serum angiotensin-converting enzyme was normal at 45 IU/L (normal range < 55 IU/L). Liver function, albumen and calcium were all normal. Chest X-ray (Fig. 13.1) showed some hilar enlargement, mainly on the left, with some upper zone infiltration. Lung function tests (forced expiratory volume in 1 s/forced vital capacity) (FEV_1/FVC) were within the predicted normal range. A tuberculin test was performed.

Progress
Because of the patient's lack of symptoms, and her partial Afro-Caribbean background, it was initially thought that sarcoidosis was the likely diagnosis. However, the tuberculin test was strongly positive (Heaf 4). A fibre-optic bronchoscopy was performed which showed no endobronchial lesion in the left upper or lingular lobe. However, washings taken from the left upper lobe were culture positive for M. tuberculosis. Conventional short-course 6-month chemo-therapy was given. The erythema nodosum was treated with the tuberculosis treatment and simple analgesia and resolved within 4 weeks. Pyrazinamide was stopped after 8 weeks when fully sensitive organisms were confirmed. The chest X-ray had virtually completely cleared by the end of treatment. Contact tracing showed no household cases with tuberculosis. Screening of all the elderly residents of the patient's workplace by chest X-ray showed no cases of tuberculosis, but a few residents had died within the previous 6 months.

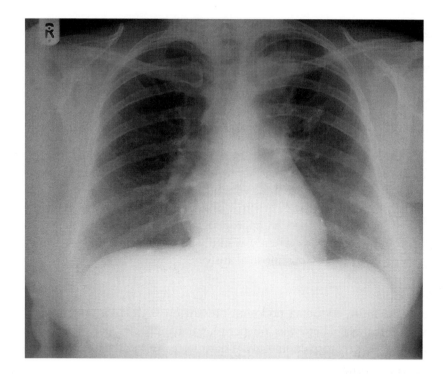

Fig. 13.1

Comment

In this case sarcoidosis was initially felt to be more likely than tuberculosis, but the strongly positive tuberculin test made that improbable. Erythema nodosum due to tuberculosis is now uncommon in developed countries, with sarcoidosis, streptococcal infections and inflammatory bowel disease all being more likely causes. The development of erythema nodosum usually accompanies tuberculin conversion and develops within 3 to 6 months of infection. No source was found in this case, and the most likely source is thought to have been one of the deceased residents who had undiagnosed tuberculosis. The erythema nodosum from tuberculosis usually settles rapidly with treatment of the tuberculosis, but simple analgesia or a non-steroidal anti-inflammatory drug (NSAID) may be needed to relieve symptoms until this occurs. Corticosteroids are rarely required.

Reference

Walgren, A. 1948: The timetable of tuberculosis. *Tubercle* **29**, 245–51.

Cross reference

Section 6B, Mediastinal lymphadenopathy

Case 14   The political refugee

Presenting complaint
A 25-year-old Indonesian man presented with a cough that had persisted for 6 months.

History of presenting complaint
The patient had come to the UK from Portugal, where he had spent 3 years as a political refugee from East Timor. Six months after his arrival in the UK he presented with a productive cough that had persisted for 6 months, and some weight loss. He had recently stopped smoking 20 cigarettes a day. He had no previous medical history.

Examination
Systemic examination was normal apart from some dullness on percussion in the left upper chest.

Tests
Chest X-ray (Fig. 14.1) showed ill-defined shadowing adjacent to the aortic knuckle and in the adjacent left upper lobe. CT scan (Fig. 14.2) showed a lobulated soft tissue density adjacent to the aortic knuckle, and some

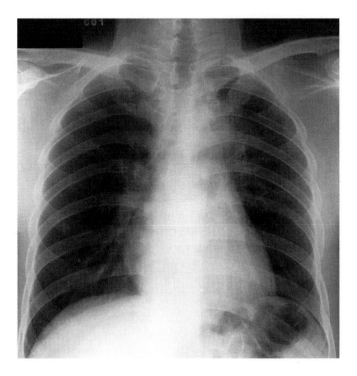

Fig. 14.1

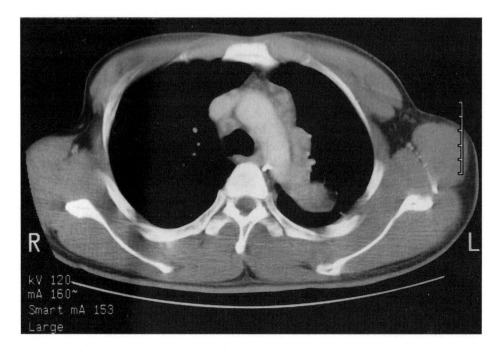

Fig. 14.2

lymphadenopathy in the pre-tracheal and subcarinal areas. Haemoglobin was 14.2 g/dL and ESR was 33 mm/h. Sputum was negative three times on microscopy for AFB. At bronchoscopy two necrotic tumour-like masses were seen at the orifices of the left upper lobe and left upper divisional bronchus (Plate 14.1). Bronchial biopsy showed inflamed bronchial mucosa with foci of necrosis and epithelioid granulomas. Bronchial washings were negative on microscopy for AFB.

Progress
The patient was started on quadruple chemotherapy with rifampicin, isoniazid, pyrazinamide and ethambutol. M. *tuberculosis* was cultured from both sputum and bronchial washings at 6 weeks, later confirmed to be fully sensitive. Pyrazinamide and ethambutol were stopped after 2 months and treatment was completed with rifampicin/isoniazid for 4 further months. The chest X-ray resolved completely and the patient gained 11 kg in weight.

Comment
Endobronchial tuberculosis is an uncommon manifestation of a common disease, and is confirmed by histological involvement of the tracheo-bronchial tree. It is reported in 10 to 40 per cent of pulmonary tuberculosis patients who have bronchoscopy (these may not be representative). Most cases are secondary either to pulmonary tuberculosis in the adjacent lung parenchyma or to endobronchial

eruption of a mediastinal or subcarinal gland. Primary cases are very uncommon. Loss of lung volume on chest X-ray may indicate development of bronchial stenosis. There is a wide variety of bronchoscopic appearances, ranging from a white gelatinous exudate to ulcerative lesions, granulomatous tumour-like lesions (as in this case) and bronchostenosis. Treatment is with standard antituberculosis chemotherapy. Dilatation, curettage and bronchial stenting may be needed for stenotic lesions, and the usefulness of corticosteroids is controversial. Bronchostenosis can occur despite adequate treatment. Complications of endobronchial tuberculosis include collapse of dependent parts of the lung, secondary pneumonia, bronchiectasis, and death by suffocation with tracheal involvement. The differential diagnosis of endobronchial tuberculosis includes sarcoidosis, tumours, fungal disease and Kaposi's sarcoma in HIV-positive patients.

Reference
Lee, J.H., Park, S.S., Lee, D.H. *et al.* 1992: Endobronchial tuberculosis: clinical and bronchoscopic features in 121 cases. *Chest* **102**, 990–4.

Case 15 The nervous secretary

Presenting complaint
A 16-year-old secretary presented with a 3-month history of intermittent shortness of breath.

History of presenting complaint
The patient had started work as a secretary in a local firm of accountants at the time when she first noticed the symptoms. Smoking was permitted in the open office area, so she was continually exposed to passive smoking, although she had never smoked herself. She noticed that she was becoming intermittently tight-chested and breathless. This tended to be worse on waking in the morning, and occasionally she had been woken up in the night by the sensation and a cough.

Past medical history
At the age of 13 years her school Heaf test was strongly positive. She had been X-rayed at the chest clinic at the time and followed up for 1 year and then discharged. From the age of 14 years she had found it very difficult to put on weight, and although her periods had started at that age, they were irregular and scanty. She had been referred to a psychiatrist, who had made a provisional diagnosis of anorexia nervosa.

Examination
Physical examination showed a thin but otherwise fit 16-year-old. No physical abnormality was found in the respiratory or cardiovascular systems or the abdomen. There was a 15-mm white rounded weal on the volar surface of the left forearm at the site of the Heaf test performed 3 years previously (Plate 15.1).

Tests
A plain chest radiograph taken in the clinic showed several small (< 2 cm in diameter) opacities at the left apex, some of which contained calcification, while others were softer with none. The patient's chest radiographs from her previous attendance at the chest clinic were found from 3 and 2 years previously. Both showed small calcified flecks at the left apex. There had been no change between the two previous films, but comparison with the current film showed that some of the softer shadowing was new. A fibre-optic bronchoscopy was performed which showed some endobronchial narrowing at the orifices of the left upper lobe and lingular lobe bronchi. Washings were taken which were negative on direct smear for AFB, but which subsequently grew fully sensitive M. tuberculosis.

Outcome

Triple therapy consisting of isoniazid, rifampicin and pyrazinamide was started the day after the bronchoscopy was performed, and was reduced to isoniazid and rifampicin after 2 months when sensitivity results were available. During therapy the patient put on 5 kg in weight and made an uneventful recovery. Her initial symptoms resolved.

Comment

The symptoms with which the patient presented were those of asthma. There is an association between tuberculosis and asthma, although in her case some of the difficulty she experienced in breathing may have been due to endobronchial tuberculosis causing airway narrowing, rather than to asthma. The scarred Heaf test site provided the clue that tuberculosis infection had been present 3 years earlier. Less than 3 per cent of white teenagers in this UK city would be expected to have a positive test. Evidence of scarring suggested a very strongly positive test, and therefore the need to exclude active tuberculosis. The chest X-ray provided the probable diagnosis, which was confirmed by obtaining bronchoscopic washings for smear and culture.

Anorexia nervosa is a differential diagnosis of tuberculosis, which should be excluded by tuberculin test and chest X-ray.

A strong case for treatment or preventive therapy could have been made at the patient's first presentation 3 years earlier. Had this been undertaken, 2 years of generalized malaise and poor health would probably have been avoided.

Case 16   The sister's father

Presenting complaint
A 65-year-old man was brought to the clinic by his daughter, a ward sister from the same hospital, with a 1-year history of weight loss.

History of presenting complaint
He had been fit with no significant past or family history of disease, and had no known contact with tuberculosis. He had smoked 20 cigarettes a day since his teens. He did not complain of cough, but had begun to feel generally tired and unable to enjoy his hobby of hill-walking. He had lost about 3 kg in weight.

Examination and tests
Physical examination showed a thin but otherwise apparently fit man with no abnormal physical findings. A chest X-ray revealed a mixture of soft and hard opacities 0.5–1.0 cm in diameter in both upper lobes (Fig. 16.1). The CT scan showed patchy alveolar shadowing in both upper lobes. There were also several rounded opacities about 2 cm diameter which were spiculated and near the pleural surface (Fig. 16.2). Three sputum samples were negative on direct smear for AAFB. A bronchoscopy showed no abnormality, and washings for cytology

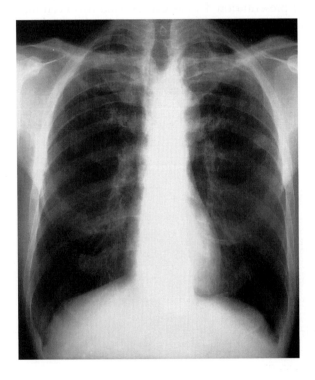

Fig. 16.1

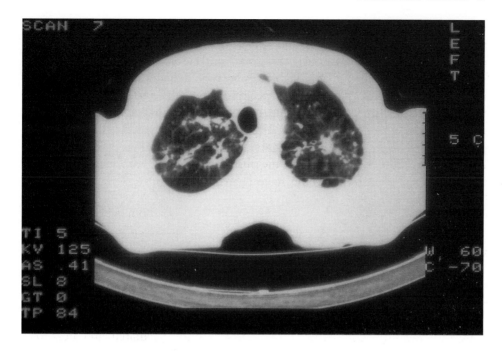

Fig. 16.2

and AAFB were also negative. A tuberculin test was strongly positive (25 mm to 10 tuberculin units).

Outcome
The patient was started on triple therapy (isoniazid, rifampicin and pyrazinamide) once the bronchoscopy had been performed. He showed some symptomatic improvement and weight gain. After 8 weeks of incubation the bronchoscopic washings grew M. *tuberculosis* that was fully sensitive to all first-line drugs. Therapy was continued for 6 months and the patient made an uneventful recovery. He said that he had stopped smoking by halfway through his treatment. The chest radiograph showed partial resolution.

Comment
This is a very characteristic patient with ongoing slowly progressive disease. He may have had previous infection or disease of which he was unaware, as was suggested by the mixture of hard and soft shadows on the chest radiograph. Bacterial counts in the sputum and bronchial washings were too low (less than 10 000 organisms/mL) to achieve smear positivity, but not too low to give culture positivity (more than 100 organisms/mL). Diagnosis was initially based on the clinical history, the positive tuberculin test and abnormalities seen on the chest radiograph, so that treatment was started before bacterial confirmation was available. The principal differential diagnosis in this patient, an older white

male smoker, was of course carcinoma of the lung. Once smear-negative sputa were obtained, a bronchoscopy and CT scan were performed in order to help exclude this diagnosis. Although this could not be entirely ruled out by these investigations, the balance of probabilities lay with a diagnosis of tuberculosis, so treatment was started. The strongly positive tuberculin test was an important factor in this decision, but it should be remembered that approximately one-third of older males in a developed country are likely to be tuberculin test positive. Had there been no clinical response to treatment and no culture confirmation after 8 weeks of therapy, further diagnostic intervention such as biopsy, or even lobectomy, would have been indicated.

SECTION 1C SMEAR-NEGATIVE, CULTURE-NEGATIVE DISEASE

Case 17 A thirsty Pakistani woman

Presenting complaint
A 64-year-old Pakistani woman was seen with a history of weight loss, thirst and cough that had persisted for 3 months.

History of presenting complaint
The patient had lived in the UK for 9 years, but had just returned from a 7-month visit to Pakistan where her symptoms had developed. She had lost 5 kg in weight and had experienced thirst for 3 months, and she also had a cough productive of mucoid sputum. She was a non-smoker and had no past history of note.

Examination
No focal signs were found in the chest, and there was no evidence of diabetic neuropathy or retinopathy. Her weight was 48 kg.

Tests
Chest X-ray showed some bilateral upper changes without cavitation (Fig. 17.1). No previous chest X-rays were available. Three sputum samples were negative for AFB on microscopy. Urinalysis showed 4+ glucose, and random blood glucose was 26 mmol/L. Haemoglobin was 11.4 g/dL, white cell count (WCC) was 7.0×10^6/mL and ESR was 38 mm/h.

Progress
The patient was started on Humulin 2 insulin bd for her diabetes, and on Rifater 4 tablets plus ethambutol 15 mg/kg (700 mg) with pyridoxine 10 mg. These drugs were continued for 2 months, by which time cultures had been reported negative. The patient gained weight rapidly, mainly because of stabilization of her diabetes, gaining 9 kg in 4 weeks. Her dosages of Rifater (5 tablets) and ethambutol (900 mg) were adjusted for weight gain. After 2 months, pyrazinamide and ethambutol were stopped. There had been some X-ray improvement after 2 months of treatment, and although bacteriological activity could not be confirmed, treatment was completed with 4 further months of rifampicin/isoniazid.

Comment
The patient's weight loss was most probably due to the onset of her diabetes. The activity of disease is only confirmed bacteriologically in about 60 to 70 per cent of cases in developed countries. Diabetics have a higher rate of tuberculosis, by a factor of two- or threefold, compared to age- and ethnically matched non-

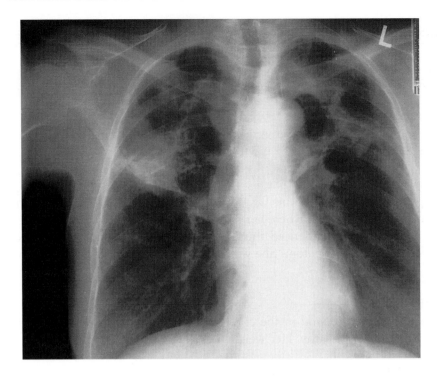

Fig. 17.1

diabetics. This was a factor in continuing treatment, and pyridoxine (10 mg) was given as prophylaxis against isoniazid peripheral neuropathy for the same reason. Clinical judgement needs to be exercised and clinical clues together with X-ray changes used to decide whether to treat. However, data from Hong Kong suggest that, in cases such as this, if treatment is not given then activity either with changing X-rays or positive cultures develops in nearly 50 per cent of cases.

Reference
Hong Kong Chest Service/Tuberculosis Research Centre Madras/British Medical Research Council. 1984: A controlled trial of 2–month, 3–month and 12–month regimens of chemotherapy for sputum smear-negative pulmonary tuberculosis. The results at 60 months. *American Review of Respiratory Diseases* **130**, 23–8.

Case 18   The asymptomatic contact

Presenting complaint
An asymptomatic 17-year-old man was seen as a household contact.

History of presenting complaint
The patient had a history of combined physical and mental handicap from birth. His mother had had smear-positive pulmonary tuberculosis 18 months earlier, when his serial tuberculin tests were negative. A further member of the family developed smear-positive tuberculosis, and he was rescreened. He had had no systemic or respiratory symptoms.

Examination
Examination showed longstanding physical and mental handicap but no respiratory signs.

Tests
The tuberculin test was strongly positive (having been negative 18 months earlier). Chest X-ray (Fig. 18.1) showed left upper zone shadowing. Liver function, haemoglobin and ESR were normal.

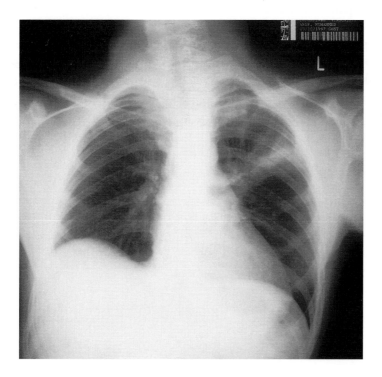

Fig. 18.1

Progress

Although the patient was asymptomatic, he was treated for tuberculosis because of the tuberculin conversion and the X-ray changes. No sputum was obtainable, and in view of his handicap it was not felt appropriate to perform bronchoscopy for washings, as both family tuberculosis cases had had fully sensitive organisms. The patient was treated with Rifater for 2 months and then with a combination of rifampicin and isoniazid for a further 4 months. Ethambutol was omitted because the family organism was fully sensitive, and mainly because the patient could not reliably undergo a visual acuity assessment and report any changes to his vision.

Comment

Tuberculosis infection in the early disease is often without symptoms and signs, even in adults. Tuberculin conversion was the only initial evidence of infection/disease. Close household contacts of sputum smear-positive respiratory cases have an incidence of tuberculous infection of up to 10 per cent, with young unvaccinated children at highest risk. Most cases are detected on the initial screening, but some tuberculin-positive adults are only detected on follow-up X-rays over a 6- to 12-month period. In children and young adults, chemo-prophylaxis for positive skin tests is appropriate in such contacts with normal X-rays. Those with abnormal X-rays have tuberculosis disease and should be treated as separate index cases.

References

British Thoracic Association. 1978: A study of a standardised contact procedure in tuberculosis. *Tubercle* **59**, 245–59.

Rose, C.E., Zerbe, G.O., Lentz, S.O. and Bailey, W.C. 1979: Establishing priority during investigation of tuberculosis contacts. *American Review of Respiratory Diseases* **119**, 603–9.

Case 19   Father to daughter

Presenting complaint
A 9-year-old Asian girl was seen with a 2-week history of cough and malaise.

History of presenting complaint
The patient had felt unwell for 2 weeks, with a dry non-productive cough and malaise, and she had felt hot and sweaty in the evenings. She was born in the UK and had not visited the Indian subcontinent. Her symptoms had not responded to 1 week of treatment with amoxycillin.

Past medical history
The patient's father had had sputum smear-positive tuberculosis some 15 months earlier, at which time she had been checked as a contact. Serial tuberculin tests had been negative.

Examination
A few crackles were heard in the left upper zone.

Tests
Chest X-ray (Fig. 19.1) showed infiltration of the left upper and mid zones. The tuberculin test was now strongly positive. The patient weighed 21.1 kg and was febrile up to 38.2°C. She was unable to produce sputum even with nebulized saline.

Progress
In view of the tuberculin change from that obtained 12 months earlier, a presumptive diagnosis of tuberculosis was made. The father's organism had been fully sensitive. Treatment with Rifater (3 tablets) and ethambutol (300 mg) was given for 2 months. This was then changed to rifampicin/isoniazid for a further 4 months. The chest X-ray showed substantial clearance over the 6-month treatment period, and the patient gained 4 kg in weight.

Comment
The likelihood of bacterial pneumonia was thought to be low because of the lack of response to antibiotics, the distribution of the X-ray changes and, in particular, the tuberculin conversion and history of tuberculosis contact. Initial and repeat screening 8 weeks after the patient's last contact had shown no evidence of tuberculosis infection. Because of this, her father, who had completed treatment about 8 months earlier, was reassessed and X-rayed, but no evidence of reactivation of tuberculosis was found. It was not considered appropriate to perform gastric washings because the organism's probable sensitivity pattern was known. It could be argued that for an organism that was probably fully sensitive ethambutol could have been omitted, but there is no

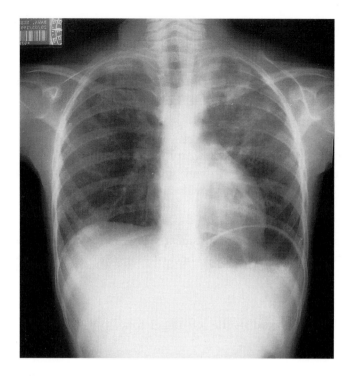

Fig. 19.1

evidence of increased toxicity of ethambutol in children, and it should be included where appropriate in the regimen.

Reference
Trebucq, A. 1997: Should ethambutol be recommended for routine treatment of tuberculosis in children? A review of the literature. *International Journal of Tuberculosis and Lung Disease* **1**, 12–15.

Cross reference
Chapter 7, Childhood disease

Case 20   A new arrival

Presenting complaint
A 25-year-old Pakistani man was seen with a 2-month history of productive cough, and weight loss of 6 kg.

History of presenting complaint
The patient had arrived in the UK from Pakistan some 15 months earlier and was a smoker. He had had a cough productive of white sputum for 2 months, with no blood or purulent material. He had lost 6 kg in weight but had not experienced night sweats, fever or chest pain. There was no past history of note.

Examination
The patient was thin, weighed 60 kg, and had no signs apart from some reduced percussion note at the right base.

Tests
Haemoglobin was 12.8 gm/dL with a mean corpuscular volume (MCV) of 63 fL. ESR was 4 mm/h and liver function tests were normal. Haemoglobin electrophoresis revealed an increased HbA_2 at 4.9 per cent showing beta-thalassaemia minor. Chest X-ray (Fig. 20.1) showed a little infiltration at the right apex, and a localized pleural collection at the right base. Three sputum samples were negative on microscopy for AFB. A pleural tap at the right base was dry and gave no fluid.

Progress
Despite the normal ESR, the presence of a small localized pleural collection and the patient's systemic symptoms suggested activity. Treatment with Rifater (5 tablets) and ethambutol (900 mg) was given for 2 months, by which time cultures were reported to be negative. Treatment was continued for a further 4 months with rifampicin/isoniazid. Over the period of treatment the patient gained 8 kg, and the basal pleural changes resolved, while those at the right apex remained largely unchanged.

Comment
The decision as to whether disease may be 'active' depends on the sum of the clinical picture, the chest X-ray and the bacteriology. Since the bacteriology results may not be available for a number of weeks, it is reasonable to embark on what is initially a trial of treatment, if there are systemic symptoms or other features which suggest disease activity, even if this is not subsequently confirmed bacteriologically. In large prospective surveys in the UK, between 25 and 35 per cent of notified tuberculosis is not bacteriologically confirmed. The response may be shown in terms of weight gain or X-ray improvement, confirming clinical

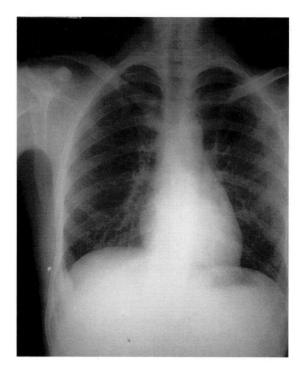

Fig. 20.1

activity even if not bacteriologically proven. There is some evidence that a 4-month regimen may be adequate for culture-negative disease, and this may have implications for resource-poor countries in particular.

References
Dutt, A.K., Dory Moers, D. and Stead, W.W. 1989: Smear- and culture-negative pulmonary tuberculosis, 4-month short-course chemotherapy. *American Review of Respiratory Diseases* **139**, 867–70.

Kumar, D., Watson, J.M., Charlett, A. *et al.* 1997: Tuberculosis in England and Wales in 1993: results of a national survey. *Thorax* **52**, 1060–6.

Case 21   The worried reporter

Presenting complaint
A 47-year-old newspaper journalist presented with a 2-month history of cough, with haemoptysis and weight loss.

History of presenting complaint
The patient had no significant previous history, but had spent some time abroad on reporting duties, principally in Eastern Europe and the Middle East. He was a heavy smoker (40 cigarettes/day), and he also drank wine and spirits regularly (approximately 50 units a week). After returning from a foreign assignment 2 months previously he had developed a chronic persistent cough with an occasional fleck of red blood mixed with the sputum. He had lost about 6 kg over the same period.

Examination and tests
Physical examination was unremarkable, but a chest X-ray showed a dense homogenous lesion in the right upper lobe (Fig. 21.1). No sputum was available, so the patient underwent fibre-optic bronchoscopy and bronchial lavage.

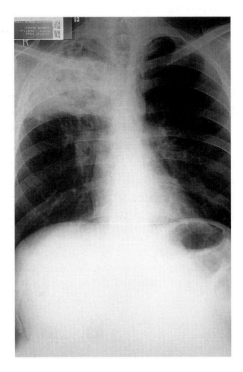

Fig. 21.1

Everything was completely normal, and washings were negative for AAFB and cytology.

A tuberculin test was strongly positive.

Outcome

The patient was started on full antituberculous chemotherapy. After 1 month of treatment he had improved symptomatically. This improvement continued at 2 months, by which time the chest X-ray had begun to show signs of clearing. Culture results remained negative after 12 weeks' incubation. The patient continued on therapy for 6 months, by which time the X-ray had almost completely resolved.

Comment

As in a previous case, the main concern of the clinician involved was that carcinoma of the lung was not being missed. A fine-needle aspirate of the lesion after the negative bronchoscopy would have been justified, but the homogeneity of the lesion meant that the entire upper lobe was apparently involved, and a negative aspiration or percutaneous needle biopsy would not have excluded the diagnosis of a carcinoma. As both the symptoms and the radiological abnormality were improving on treatment, further diagnostic tests were not requested. In effect, the trial of therapy used on this patient was in itself a diagnostic test. The surprising aspect of this case was the extent of the radiographic disease (the whole of the right upper lobe was affected) in the absence of bacteriological confirmation of diagnosis. The possibility remains that the lung lesion represented an infection from some other organism, which responded slowly to antituberculous chemotherapy, but antibody titres for other possible infectious causes such as viruses or mycoplasma remained low. The time-course of development and cure of disease was characteristic of tuberculosis, and the organism is notoriously difficult to culture and identify. Laboratory error resulting from overenthusiasm about eliminating contaminants may sometimes lead to a false-negative culture, as M. tuberculosis can be killed off by anti-contamination measures.

The patient resumed some part-time work after a few weeks of treatment, and resumed full-time employment after 3 months.

Case 22   Right second time (probably)

Presenting complaint

A 60-year-old man presented with a history of several months of cough, weight loss and malaise.

Tests

Physical examination was unremarkable, but a chest X-ray showed upper lobe shadowing (Fig. 22.1) with apparent cavitation. A bronchoscopy showed no abnormality, and washings were negative for AFB. A Mantoux test was very strongly positive.

Progress

In view of the probability of tuberculosis, the patient was started on triple therapy (isoniazid, rifampicin and pyrazinamide). Two months later there had been little clinical progress, and the cultures from bronchoscopy showed no growth. However, antituberculous chemotherapy was continued for a full 6 months. The chest radiograph showed some improvement during this time, but there was no weight gain. *Aspergillus* precipitins were strongly positive. A CT scan confirmed upper lobe fibrosis and cavitation and bronchiectasis. Within this cavity a solid body, probably an aspergilloma, was observed.

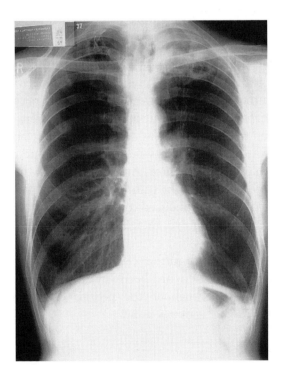

Fig. 22.1

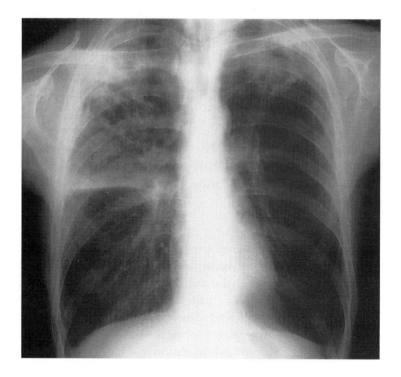

Fig. 22.2

The patient was followed up intermittently following cessation of tuberculosis therapy, but he continued to complain of cough and a little haemoptysis. Two years after the end of his treatment he presented with further malaise and loss of 6 kg in weight in the preceding 6 weeks. A chest X-ray showed extensive shadowing on the right and some on the left (Fig. 22.2). Bronchoscopy was again performed and found to be normal. Washings for AFB were again negative. The patient was put back on triple therapy and supervised more closely with home visits by the tuberculosis health visitor. At 1-month follow-up he was clinically much improved, with a 2-kg weight gain and improvement of his chest X-ray. After 2 months his therapy was reduced to two drugs (isoniazid and rifampicin) and his X-ray continued to improve. Bronchial washings were again negative for AFB.

In view of the possibility of a further relapse, treatment was continued for a full 12 months. By this time there had been virtually complete resolution of the chest X-ray (Fig. 22.3) Throughout the periods of treatment the patient continued to smoke 20–30 cigarettes a day.

Comment

At no point was the diagnosis of tuberculosis confirmed in this patient. The relatively slight abnormalities on the chest X-rays at the first episode and the

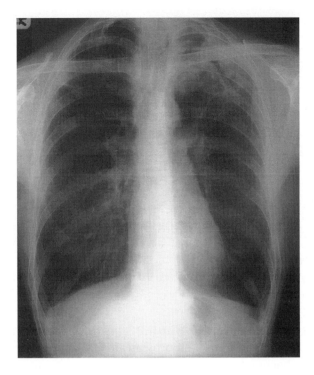

Fig. 22.3

finding of a probable aspergilloma on CT scanning indicate that active tuberculosis was probably not present during the first episode of treatment. However, the very extensive chest X-ray changes at the start of the second episode and the response to treatment make the diagnosis during this second episode more likely, but by no means certain. It may seem odd that the treatment given for the first episode did not prevent the occurrence of the second episode. However, compliance during the first episode was uncertain.

By the time culture results were available the second time, the patient was showing clinical and radiographic improvement, so continuation of treatment was logical. Had this not been the case, further investigation – including biopsy of the radiographic abnormalities – would have been indicated.

Approximately 25 per cent of pulmonary tuberculosis remains unconfirmed bacteriologically, the diagnosis being made on clinical grounds, including response to treatment.

Management of adverse drug reactions

Case 23   A man with bleeding gums

Presenting complaint
A 60-year-old man presented with a history of gum bleeding for 3 days while he was on antituberculosis treatment.

History of presenting complaint
The patient had been well until 5 months previously, when he was admitted for investigation of haemoptysis and weight loss. Chest X-rays after admission showed a shadow in the right upper zone. Sputum smear examination for AFB was negative. Fibre-optic bronchoscopy was performed, which showed no endobronchial lesion. Bronchial aspirate for AFB was smear positive. The patient was put on antituberculosis treatment with isoniazid, rifampicin, pyrazinamide and ethambutol. He made good clinical and radiological progress in response to treatment, and the regimen was changed to isoniazid and rifampicin at 3 months. The culture and sensitivity test results for the bronchial aspirate revealed M. tuberculosis sensitive to first-line drugs.

Five months after the start of treatment, the patient began to notice gum bleeding as well as petechiae over the upper part of the body. He attended the chest clinic on the third day. Drug-induced thrombocytopenia was suspected, and treatment was immediately withheld. The patient was admitted to hospital for further investigation.

Past medical history
There was no past medical history of blood disorder. The patient had no previous history of tuberculosis, nor did he have any history of antituberculosis treatment.

Examination
Physical examination revealed bleeding gums and a haematoma over the right side of the upper surface of the tongue. There were also multiple petechiae over the upper part of the body. The patient was afebrile. No lymph nodes were

palpable, and examination of the chest and cardiovascular system did not reveal any abnormalities. No signs of enlarged liver or spleen were detected on examination of the abdomen.

Tests

An examination of the complete blood profile confirmed a reduced platelet count of $14 \times 10^9/L$. The haemoglobin level and platelet count were normal. Blood samples for antinuclear factor and rheumatoid factors were negative.

Outcome

All of the drugs were omitted and the patient received a platelet concentrate transfusion. Within 1 week his platelet count had returned to normal. Because rifampicin-induced thrombocytopenia was suspected, treatment was restarted with isoniazid, ethambutol and pyrazinamide. The patient received the latter three drugs for a further 4 months and made an uneventful recovery. He was advised against taking rifampicin for the rest of his life.

Comment

Numerous examples of rifampicin-induced thrombocytopenia have been documented in the literature, and a number of cases were observed during high-dose intermittent treatment. The complication is rare when the drug is given in small doses. A few cases of thrombocytopenia have occurred after administration of rifampicin following an interruption of therapy. The return of the platelet count to normal after cessation of administration of the drug in our patient confirmed the diagnosis.

The thrombocytopenia might be explained by the presence of IgG and IgM antibodies to rifampicin. These antibodies are capable of fixing complement to the platelets in the presence of rifampicin. It is believed that the drug may act as a hapten and combine with macromolecules in the plasma which become antigenic. Antibodies are produced against the drug which, when readministered, forms a hapten–antibody complex which is absorbed onto the surface of the platelet and binds to complement, so causing destruction of the platelet.

The development of anti-rifampicin antibodies depends on both the size of the dose given and the rhythm of rifampicin administration. No relationship has been shown between the duration of treatment and the development of rifampicin-dependent antibodies. The lower incidence of the thrombocytopenia, including the effect of rifampicin, during daily dosages as compared to intermittent regimens might possibly be attributed to the presence of neutralizing antibodies formed during continuous treatment. The antibody complex is believed to be removed continuously without causing an allergic reaction.

Patients with adverse risk factors

Case 24   The feverish Asian

Presenting complaint
A 63-year-old Asian woman was seen with fever and bilateral cervical lymphadenopathy.

History of presenting complaint
The glands had been swollen for 4–6 weeks and were non-tender, but were associated with evening fever. There had been no discharge from the glands, and there was no overlying erythema.

Past medical history
Two years earlier the patient had presented with ascites and splenomegaly. Ultrasound confirmed these findings, and further investigations showed micro-nodular cirrhosis on biopsy, while virology showed the patient to be hepatitis C antibody positive at high titre. There was evidence of oesophageal varices, a blood picture of hypersplenism, and deranged coagulation. For 4 months the patient had been on the active waiting-list for liver transplant.

Examination
There was bilateral cervical lymphadenopathy (right greater than left) with glands up to 2 cm in diameter in the anterior triangles. Ascites and splenomegaly were present. The patient's weight was 40 kg.

Tests
A gland biopsy showed large areas of caseation with several tuberculoid granulomata, of which part was sent for culture. Haemoglobin was 11.2 g/dL. The white cell count was 1.8×10^6/mL and the platelet count was 65×10^9/mL. ESR was 110 mm/h, bilirubin was 33 mmol/L, alanine aminotransferase (ALT)

was 37 IU/L, globulin was 51 g/L and albumen was 29 g/L. Chest X-ray was normal.

Progress
On confirmation of tuberculosis, the transplant centre removed the patient from the active waiting-list.

Treatment was commenced with Rifater (4 tablets, each containing 120 mg rifampicin, 50 mg of isoniazid and 300 mg pyrazinamide) giving a total dose of 480 mg rifampicin, 200 mg isoniazid and 1200 mg pyrazinamide, together with 600 mg ethambutol and 10 mg pyridoxine.

Liver function tests were monitored three times weekly for the first 2 weeks, and then twice weekly for a further 2 weeks. There was no change in the liver function tests, and the patient's low-grade fever resolved. She was allowed home after 4 weeks of monitoring, having weekly liver function tests. After 8 weeks of treatment she had gained 5 kg in weight, the fever had resolved and the glands were substantially smaller. Cultures were reported to be negative. Ethambutol and pyrazinamide were stopped, and treatment continued for a further 4 months with Rifinah 150 (3 tablets; rifampicin 450 mg, isoniazid 300 mg) and pyridoxine. Liver function was tested every 2 weeks in the third month of treatment and then monthly until completion. After 6 months the glands had resolved, the patient weighed 48 kg, and treatment was stopped. Liver function had not altered significantly throughout the 6-month treatment period. The patient was reinstated on the active transplant list, but died several months later of liver failure without a donor having been found.

Comment
This patient had severe liver disease and tuberculosis. Her only chance of long-term survival was to have adequate treatment of her tuberculosis to allow her to go back on to the active transplant list. The options were either to give full short-course chemotherapy, or to give a weaker regimen with a lower risk of hepatic toxicity, e.g. isoniazid/ethambutol for 15–18 months, although this would take much longer to achieve cure. Full treatment was started as an in-patient with very regular monitoring, and the frequency of monitoring was gradually reduced when there were no reactions. The patient's liver function did not alter significantly throughout the course of treatment.

Reference
Ormerod, L.P., Skinner, C. and Wales, J.M. 1996: Hepatotoxicity of anti-tuberculosis drugs. *Thorax* **51**, 111–13.

Case 25   The alcoholic with weight loss

Presenting complaint
A 44-year-old female alcoholic presented with weight loss.

History of presenting complaint
The patient's usual alcohol consumption rate was in excess of 10 units/day, and she had lost more than 10 kg during the preceding 4 months. She currently weighed 37.4 kg, and she smoked 20 cigarettes a day and had a productive cough.

Previous medical history
The patient had a history of alcoholism for over 10 years but no other illnesses, and no known tuberculosis contact.

Examination
The patient was thin, there was no clubbing, and scattered crackles were present in the upper zones bilaterally. Neither hepatomegaly nor stigmata of chronic liver disease were present. Fever was present (up to 39.5°C).

Tests
Chest X-ray showed extensive bilateral cavitatory disease (Fig. 25.1) and sputum was 3+ positive for AFB. Haemoglobin was 8.9 g/dL, with an MCV of 112 fL (normal range 80–98 fL). Sodium was 129 mmol/L, urea was 2.0 mmol/L, ALT was 93 U/L and serum albumen was 27 g/L. Abdominal X-ray showed no pancreatic calcification.

Progress
Triple therapy was commenced as an in-patient with weekly liver function monitoring. Prednisolone (50 mg/day) was added after 1 week because of continued fever, poor appetite, and the extent of disease. The fever resolved after 3 weeks, but there was no weight gain. All antituberculosis drugs were being given under direct supervision. Thiamine (100 mg), pyridoxine (10 mg) and other B vitamins had been given since the start of treatment. Thyroid function was normal. Small-bowel barium studies showed no evidence of enteric tuberculosis. Blood levels of rifampicin were satisfactory. However, tests of pancreatic function were abnormal, with a pancreolauryl test showing only 9 per cent absorption (normal range 20 per cent or greater). Pancreatic supplements as Creon (20 000 units, three times daily) were added, and a slow weight gain of 0.5 kg per week was observed. Liver function was tested fortnightly after the first month. Cultures confirmed M. tuberculosis that was fully sensitive to all first-line drugs. Inhaled bronchodilator (terbutaline) was added because of severe airflow obstruction (FEV_1 1.1/2.65 L, predicted value 2.69/3.29 L. Steroids were tailed down to zero. Treatment was switched from daily to three times weekly with

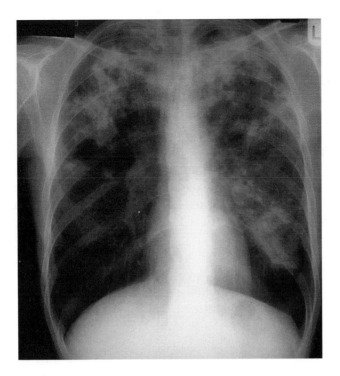

Fig. 25.1

appropriate dosage adjustments as an out-patient by directly observed therapy (DOT), and the pyrazinamide was stopped after 2 months. On completion of treatment the patient had gained 9 kg, but considerable X-ray changes persisted, although most cavities had closed.

Comment
The extensive smear-positive disease in an alcoholic was treated with standard therapy, but with regular liver function monitoring because of pre-existing liver disease. The failure to gain weight despite adequate therapy together with steroids caused concern. Small-bowel disease and failure to absorb rifampicin were excluded. Pancreatic malabsorption was demonstrated, although no calcification was seen on plain X-ray. Treatment was given under supervision throughout, initially in hospital and then as three times weekly DOT (as should be conducted with such patients and others who are likely to be non-compliant with medication). Pyridoxine was also given because of the increased likelihood of isoniazid neuropathy in alcoholics.

Reference
Ormerod L.P., Skinner, C. and Wales, J.M. 1996: Hepatotoxicity of anti-tuberculosis drugs. *Thorax* **51**, 111–13.

Case 26 A jaundiced man with weight loss; all was not what it seemed

Presenting complaint
A 62-year-old white man was admitted with a history of profound weight loss and jaundice.

History of presenting complaint
In the 3 months prior to admission the patient had lost over 20 kg in weight and had developed malaise and anorexia and mild sweats. In the month prior to admission he had developed pruritis, followed by jaundice and dark urine. He smoked 15 cigarettes a day but was a non-drinker. He had a morning cough productive of mucoid sputum.

Past medical history
The patient had had mild chronic obstructive pulmonary disease (COPD) related to his smoking in the past.

Examination
He was significantly jaundiced, with scratch marks but with no stigmata of chronic liver disease. There was no hepatomegaly or palpable gall bladder.

Tests
The patient's haemoglobin was 11.2g/dL normochromic with an ESR of 76 mm/ h. Bilirubin was 214 mmol/L, alkaline phosphatase was 1207 IU/L (normal range < 135 IU/L), aspartate transaminase (AST) was 991 IU/L (normal range < 56 IU/L), with an albumen level of 31 g/L. Prothrombin time was prolonged at 46 s (normal value 16 s), and this did not improve with vitamin K treatment. Ultrasound of the abdomen showed mild hepatomegaly, but no dilated intra- or extra-hepatic ducts and no pancreatic mass. Virology for hepatitis A and B was negative. There was a low-grade fever.

Progress
The initial diagnosis had been of pancreatic carcinoma, but when no intra- or extra-hepatic biliary obstruction was found, alternative diagnoses were sought. The jaundice was of a mixed obstructive/hepatitic type. Auto-antibodies (including antimitochondrial types) were negative. In view of the cough, a chest X-ray (Fig. 26.1) was performed which showed extensive soft shadowing throughout all zones. A previous chest X-ray was found from 5 years earlier (Fig. 26.2) which showed a calcified scar at the right apex only. Sputum when examined for AFB was 3+ positive on microscopy. A diagnosis of tuberculous bronchopneumonia was made. The patient's coagulation prevented a liver biopsy for diagnosis, and despite his deranged liver funtion test it was felt that his extensive respiratory disease required full antituberculosis treatment.

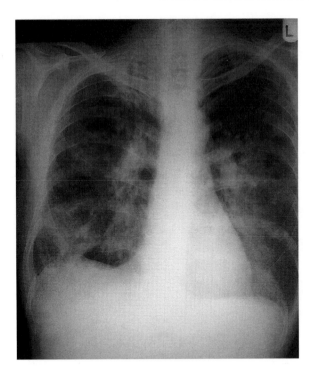

Fig. 26.1

Rifampicin, isoniazid, pyrazinamide and ethambutol at full dosage were commenced together with prednisolone (30 mg daily). Three-times-weekly liver function tests were monitored initially.

Over the next 8 weeks the patient and his liver function improved rapidly. By 8 weeks his chest X-ray had returned to the appearances seen in Fig. 26.2, and his liver function showed only an alkaline phosphatase of 186 IU/L. Sputum was culture positive for fully sensitive M. tuberculosis. Steroids were tailed off after 8 weeks, and rifampicin/isoniazid were given for a further 4 months.

Comment

Despite the extent of the chest X-ray changes, respiratory symptoms were few and were attributed to the patient's smoking. It was assumed from his response to antituberculosis drugs that he had a more disseminated tuberculosis infection with a tuberculous hepatitis, but this could not be confirmed by biopsy because of the poor coagulation. There was concern about giving rifampicin, isoniazid and pyrazinamide in the presence of very abnormal liver function, as all three drugs are potentially hepatotoxic. However, the risk/benefit analysis was that the patient's risk of dying of tuberculosis was very high without full treatment, that the jaundice was probably related to liver involvement in disseminated tuberculosis, and that the incidence of hepatitis on treatment is only of the order

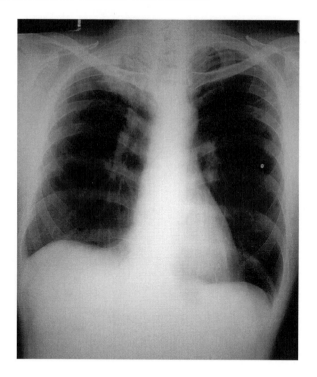

Fig. 26.2

of 3 per cent, although it may possibly be higher in an older man. Corticosteroids were given because of the patient's general condition, the extent of his pulmonary disease, and to attempt to reduce the likelihood of a drug-induced hepatitis.

Cross reference
Chapter 1, Section 1A, Smear-positive, culture-positive disease

SECTION 3B RENAL FAILURE

Case 27 Lassitude and frequency

Presenting complaint
A 62-year-old white man was referred with lassitude, weight loss of 7 kg and increasing urinary frequency.

History of presenting complaint
The patient had been well with no prior medical history until 4 months previously. Progressive lassitude had developed together with gradual weight loss of 7 kg. Over the same period of time he had had increasing nocturia and frequency, with the latter at least hourly during the day and nocturia every 1–2 h. There had been no dysuria or visible haematuria.

Examination
Rectal examination showed a small hard prostate. The patient was rather pale.

Tests
Ultrasound examination of the kidneys showed a small scarred left kidney (6.5 cm) and a dilated right ureter and hydronephrosis. ESR was 76 mm/h. A midstream specimen of urine (MSSU) showed a sterile pyuria. Blood urea was 23 mmol/L and creatinine was 640 mmol/L. An urgent cystoscopy was performed which showed a very inflamed bladder with a maximum capacity of 50 mL. The ureteric orifices could not be identified for stenting. Biopsies were taken for histology and AFB culture, and urine was sent for tuberculosis culture. The chest X-ray was normal. The bladder biopsy showed multiple caseating granulomata with a destroyed mucosal lining and AFB visible on microscopy in the bladder wall (Plate 27.1). Prostatic biopsy also showed granulomata.

Progress
The patient was commenced on Rifater and prednisolone (50 mg/day) because of the ureteric involvement. He was catheterized and a right nephrostomy was performed. After 8 days he became frankly jaundiced (bilirubin 35 mmol/L; ALT 573 IU/L), and antituberculosis drugs were stopped.

After 10 days liver function had returned to normal pre-treatment levels. Isoniazid was introduced initially in increasing dosages with ciprofloxacin 750 mg bd as cover. Streptomycin and ethambutol were contraindicated with a creatinine level still in excess of 500 mmol/L. Liver function remained normal as isoniazid and then rifampicin were serially reintroduced. Right ureteric stenting was now possible. The bladder wall and urine grew M. *tuberculosis* that was fully sensitive to antituberculosis drugs. Ciprofloxacin (750 mg bd) was given with rifampicin (600 mg) and isoniazid (300 mg) for 2 months. Creatinine had fallen to 271 mmol/L by that stage. Ciprofloxacin was then stopped and rifampicin/isoniazid were given for a further 7 months. Urea was 12.8 mmol/L and creatinine was 210 mmol/L on completion of treatment. A detailed urological assessment is planned, and if bladder capacity remains low an ileo-cystoplasty to increase bladder capacity will be performed.

Comments

The onset of tuberculous renal disease is insidious, and there can be substantial loss of kidney function before presentation due either to direct renal damage or obstructive uropathy from seeding into the ureter with subsequent obstruction. Frequency due to a markedly reduced bladder capacity from inflammation and fibrosis can occur, as in the present case. The finding of a sterile pyuria should always raise the possibility of renal tuberculosis and cause early-morning urine specimens to be sent for AFB culture. Standard treatment can be given for renal disease, with pyridoxine because of the increased risk of neuropathy. Ethambutol should be used with considerable caution in renal impairment, with much reduced dosages and serum-level monitoring.

Reference

Gow, J.G. and Barbosa, S. 1984: Genitourinary tuberculosis. A study of 1117 cases over a period of 43 years. *British Journal of Urology* **56**, 449–55.

Cross references

Chapter 2, Management of adverse drug reactions; Chapter 3, Patients with adverse risk factors

Case 28   Acute renal failure in a diabetic patient

Presenting complaint
A 54-year-old Pakistani man was seen with a 6-week history of pyrexia and weight loss, and dyspnoea for 2 weeks.

History of presenting complaint
The patient had first come to the UK in 1966, and had lived in Pakistan between 1986 and 1991, returning 4 years before his presentation. He had complained of weight loss with some fever for 6 weeks, had been diagnosed as a maturity-onset diabetic 2 weeks before arrival at the hospital, but had been becoming dyspnoeic on effort during those 2 weeks.

Examination
There was no evidence of retinopathy or neuropathy. The patient was febrile at 38°C with a sinus tachycardia but no focal signs.

Tests
Chest X-ray showed bilateral hazy shadowing (Fig. 28.1). Haemoglobin was 13.8 g/dL, ESR was 17 mm/h, and glucose was 8.9 mmol/L. Albumen was low at 25 g/L, alkaline phosphatase was 710 IU/mL, and gamma-glutamyl transferase (gamma-GT) was 663 IU/L. Urea was 21.4 mmol/L and creatinine was 226 mmol/L. Ultrasound showed an enlarged but uniform liver, with no ascites or intra-abdominal nodes and normal renal size. Urinalysis showed 2+ protein.

Progress
The patient was treated with amoxycillin and erythromycin for a few days while investigations were performed, but in view of his non-response and the above results he was started on Rifater and prednisolone (30 mg/day) after early-morning urine (EMU) and sputum had been sent for AFB culture. On the second day after starting treatment his urea level was 37.5 mmol/L and creatinine was 447 mmol/L, and the following day the corresponding values were 48 and 726 mmol/L, respectively. Antinuclear cytoplasmic antibody (ANCA) and anti-glomerular basement membrane (GBM) antibodies were negative. The patient was transferred to the renal physicians for haemodialysis and renal biopsy. The renal biopsy (Plate 28.1) showed eight normal glomeruli but marked interstitial inflammation, and in one area the biopsy had gone through the wall of an abscess. Significant numbers of AFB were seen. Treatment with Rifater and prednisolone was continued. Haemodialysis was needed for about 10 days. The liver function tests also progressively improved. Pyridoxine was given as prophylaxis for isoniazid neuropathy because of diabetes and renal failure. Urine and sputum were both culture positive for fully sensitive *M. tuberculosis*. Pyrazinamide was stopped after 2 months when the chest X-ray had largely

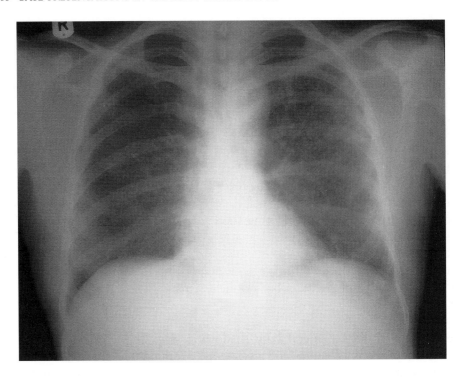

Fig. 28.1

cleared. Steroids were tailed off over 4 months. Treatment was completed with rifampicin/isoniazid for 4 months. At the completion of treatment the patient had gained 13 kg in weight, and liver function and renal function were normal.

Comment
Tuberculous interstitial nephritis can occur on its own, or more commonly as part of a more disseminated tuberculosis illness, as in the present case. Standard dosages of rifampicin, isoniazid and pyrazinamide can be given in renal impairment. Here the acute renal failure was due to the disease and not the treatment. Steroids are indicated in tuberculous interstitial nephritis to suppress inflammatory reactions and to allow a more rapid recovery of renal function.

Reference
Morgan, S.H., Eastwood, J.B. and Baker, L.R.I. 1990: TB interstitial nephritis – the tip of the iceberg? *Tubercle* **71**, 5–6.

SECTION 3C PREGNANCY

Case 29 Pregnancy during treatment

Presenting complaint
A 21-year-old Indian woman, born in the UK, was seen as a contact of a family case (smear-negative, culture-positive respiratory disease). She had no symptoms.

History of presenting complaint
The patient had been seen as a tuberculosis contact 4 years earlier with normal chest X-ray and a tuberculin test that was grade 1 positive, consistent with BCG history.

Examination
The patient appeared normal. Her weight was 53 kg.

Tests
Chest X-ray showed early infiltration in the right apex. The tuberculin test was now strongly positive (Heaf grade 4). Routine blood tests were normal.

Progress
Although the patient was asymptomatic, because of the tuberculin conversion since her previous test, and the early infiltration of the apex, treatment was given. Rifater (5 tablets daily) was given for 2 months. This was changed to a rifampicin/isoniazid combination after 2 months. In month 3 there was some nausea. Liver function tests were normal, but a pregnancy test was positive. Treatment with rifampicin/isoniazid was continued for a total of 6 months. The pregnancy was completed uneventfully. Chest X-ray with lead-apron shielding of the fetus at 20 weeks' gestation showed the right apical infiltration to have resolved.

Comment
Early disease is often asymptomatic and may show few signs. Only tuberculin conversion may be found. With apical shadowing this can be subtle, and it may be partially obscured by the anterior first and second ribs. An apical lordotic view may be required if there is doubt. Standard short-course treatment was given. The patient became pregnant during the treatment, but the latter was continued uninterrupted. The first-line drugs rifampicin, isoniazid, pyrazinamide and ethambutol are not teratogenic and can be given in pregnancy. Streptomycin and other aminoglycosides should be avoided in pregnancy because of the risk of ototoxicity to the fetus. Ethionamide and prothionamide may be teratogenic and should be avoided in pregnancy. If a mother has active

tuberculosis, the risk of miscarriage due to the disease is much higher than any risk from the drug treatment, so standard treatment should be given.

If the mother is smear positive within a few weeks of birth, the neonate should be given isoniazid primary prophylaxis (5 mg/kg), but should not be separated from the mother.

Case 30   The swelling over the hip

Presenting complaint
A 20-year-old Asian woman was seen with a painful swelling over the left hip.

History of presenting complaint
The patient had been in the UK for 1 year and had had a swelling above the left hip for 4 months and discomfort for 3 months. At the time that she was seen she was also 14 weeks pregnant. There was no past medical history of note.

Examination
There was a fluctuant swelling above the left hip laterally at the level of the anterior superior iliac spine.

Tests
An X-ray (with fetal protection) showed no bony lesion in the hemipelvis or hip. ESR was 20 mm/h.

Progress
The lesion was aspirated and pus obtained which was negative on standard culture and on microscopy for AFB. A few weeks later a discharging sinus developed at the aspiration site and a skin biopsy taken from this by the patient's family doctor showed multiple granulomata. She was then seen by the chest service, and was started on antituberculous therapy with rifampicin, isoniazid and pyrazinamide as a combination tablet (Rifater). The original pus aspirated was reported to be positive on culture for fully sensitive M. tuberculosis. The patient was seen 3 weeks later with vomiting and jaundice, with a bilirubin level of 51 mmol/L and ALT of 132 IU/L. Her family doctor, instead of continuing Rifater (4 tablets), because this was not on his computer database, had given Rifinah 300 (4 tablets) (rifampicin 1200 mg and isoniazid 600 mg daily). At least it was known that pyrazinamide was not causing the hepatitis! The medication was stopped until the patient's liver function returned to normal, and then Rifater (4 tablets daily) was reintroduced without problems. Her progress was then uneventful. Pyrazinamide was dropped after 2 months of correct treatment, and rifampicin and isoniazid (in correct dosages) were given for a further 4 months. The sinus healed after 2 months, and the patient delivered a normal baby boy 2 months before completing treatment.

Comment
The clinical site appears to have been a soft-tissue abscess without underlying bony involvement, but radiology was limited because of the patient's pregnancy. The only problem during treatment was an iatrogenic drug-induced hepatitis. Because the triple combination tablet Rifater was not on a computerized

prescribing database, the nearest rifampicin-containing combination was selected instead, and this led to overdose of both rifampicin and isoniazid, causing dose-related hepatitis. Fortunately there were no long-term complications for either the mother or her child. Care is needed when writing about and dispensing antituberculosis drugs. In some countries the similarities between the names rifampicin and those of rifampicin-containing combinations can lead to confusion and incorrect treatment.

Cross reference
Chapter 2, Management of adverse drug reactions

Drug
resistance

Case 31   It runs in the family

Presenting complaint
A 15-year-old Asian girl was seen with a history of cough, sputum and nocturnal fever.

History of presenting complaint
The cough/sputum had been present for 2 months and the nocturnal fever for 1 month. There had been some weight loss but no haemoptysis.

Past medical history
The patient had been seen 15 months earlier as a contact of an older brother with smear-positive tuberculosis which was resistant to isoniazid and strepto-mycin. Her X-rays had been clear and her tuberculin tests appropriate for her vaccination history.

Examination
The patient was thin at 34.7 kg, and febrile at 38.2°C, with a few crackles in the left upper zone.

Tests
Chest X-ray (Fig. 31.1) showed left upper zone infiltration with early cavitation. Haemoglobin was 9.5 g/dL, with an MCV of 67 fL and an ESR of 92 mm/h. Haemoglobin electrophoresis showed the patient to be HbDD homozygous. Sputum tests showed 3+ smear positivity.

Progress
The patient was admitted to a single side-ward and started treatment on ethambutol 500 mg, rifampicin 450 mg and pyrazinamide 1.5 g daily, isoniazid and streptomycin resistance being assumed. Continuing fever led to the introduction of steroids after 2 weeks. After 4 weeks the patient had gained 3 kg in weight and was afebrile. She was discharged on three times weekly supervised DOT with rifampicin 600 mg (15 mg/kg), pyrazinamide 2.0 g (50 mg/kg) and

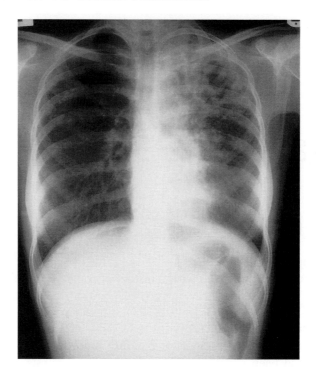

Fig. 31.1

ethambutol 900 mg (25 mg/kg). Cultures were positive at 5 weeks, and M. *tuberculosis* sensitive to rifampicin, ethambutol and pyrazinamide but highly resistant to isoniazid and streptomycin was confirmed. Pyrazinamide was stopped at 2 months, and rifampicin and ethambutol were continued for a further 7 months by three times weekly supervised DOT. Sputum cultures were negative at 2 months. There was substantial X-ray clearance during treatment, with only minimal residual left upper zone scarring. The patient gained 8.8 kg in weight during treatment. Follow-up for 2 years after cessation of treatment showed no relapse.

Comment
Because of the history of contact and the fact that the drug-resistance profile of the likely organism was known, treatment was straightforward but was given fully supervised in order to prevent the possible emergence of any additional drug resistance. If isolated isoniazid resistance is known before treatment is started, a supervised regimen consisting of 2 months' rifampicin, pyrazinamide, streptomycin and ethambutol, followed by 7 months' rifampicin and ethambutol has been shown to be effective (Babu Swai *et al.*, 1988). Here streptomycin was not given because of the presumed, and subsequently confirmed, resistance to the drug. The more usual situation is for isoniazid resistance to be shown from

initial cultures during treatment. Because of higher rates of isoniazid resistance in ethnic minority groups, those who are HIV-positive and those with a previous history of treatment, a four-drug initial combination (rifampicin, isoniazid, pyrazinamide and ethambutol) (HRZE) should be given and continued either for 2 months or for longer if cultures have been obtained and sensitivity results are outstanding. Pyrazinamide and ethambutol can then be stopped for fully sensitive organisms. If isoniazid resistance is found, in effect an initial phase of three drugs (rifampicin, pyrazinamide and ethambutol) (RZE) has been given. The pyrazinamide can be stopped and rifampicin/ethambutol (RE) continued for between 7 and 10 months.

Reference
Babu Swai, O., Alnoch, J.A., Githui, W.A. *et al.* 1988: Controlled clinical trial of a regimen of 2 durations for the treatment of isoniazid resistant tuberculosis. *Tubercle* **69**, 5–11.

Case 32 Too many vitamins may not be good for you

Presenting complaint
A 28-year-old white man was seen with weight loss, fever and haemoptysis.

History of presenting complaint
The patient had been working on a Spanish island for 2 years in the tourist industry, and had felt unwell for nearly a year. He had lost over 10 kg in weight, and had had fever with night sweats for 2 months, and haemoptysis for 1 month, the increasing severity of which caused him to present. He had not had BCG vaccination, and there was no family history of tuberculosis. A chambermaid at the apartment complex had had tuberculosis 1 year earlier. There was no past history of note.

Tests
A chest X-ray showed extensive cavitatory disease in both upper lobes (Fig. 32.1). Sputum was positive on microscopy for AFB.

Progress
In the Spanish hospital the patient was started on Rifater (5 tablets) and ethambutol (1100 mg), plus pyridoxine (300 mg) daily. Sputum taken at the

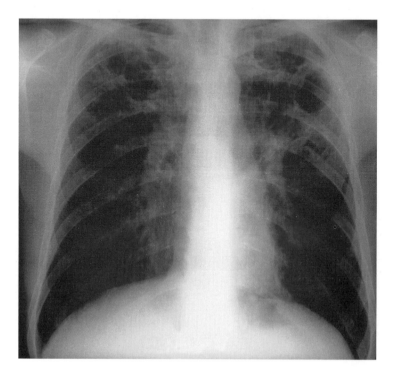

Fig. 32.1

commencement of treatment was later culture positive and reported to be fully sensitive to all first-line drugs. Because the patient remained sputum smear positive after 2 weeks of treatment he was not allowed to leave hospital, and it was only after 7 weeks that he was discharged and returned to the UK. His weight was 73 kg, his drug dosages were increased to Rifater 6 tablets and ethambutol 1200 mg, and the pyridoxine was stopped. At this stage his sputum was smear negative. Pyrazinamide was stopped after 2 months of treatment, with rifampicin and isoniazid continued as Rifinah 300 (2 tablets), the ethambutol being stopped 4 weeks later when the patient's initial sensitivity results were received from Spain. His sputum at 2 months was eventually culture positive after 9 weeks, and grew only slowly on subculture but was found to be highly resistant to isoniazid. Treatment was switched to rifampicin and ethambutol for a further 5 months.

Sputum was culture negative at the end of treatment. The patient had suffered considerable lung damage, with an FEV_1 of 2.45/3.50 L (predicted value = 4.71/5.81 L).

Comment
It was unjustified to keep the patient in hospital after 2 weeks, even though he was still smear positive, as 2 weeks of treatment with rifampicin/isoniazid renders a person non-infectious even if bacilli can still be observed in the sputum. The grossly excessive dose of pyridoxine (vitamin B_6) was stopped immediately in the UK, as pyridoxine antagonizes isoniazid on a milligram-for-milligram basis. The 300 mg dose of vitamin B_6 had completely antagonized the dose of isoniazid he had received (10 mg daily is ample to prevent peripheral neuropathy). The finding of isoniazid resistance after 7 weeks of therapy was unexpected, but was thought to be entirely due to the above physician error. The patient had received combination tablets throughout, making accidental or deliberate monotherapy with isoniazid impossible, and his compliance in the UK had been entirely satisfactory during monitoring. Continuation therapy was therefore prolonged.

Because of the extensive lung involvement the patient was left with substantial lung damage.

Reference
Jindani, A., Aber, V.R., Edwards, E.A. and Mitchison, D.A. 1980: The early bactericidal activity of drugs in patients with pulmonary tuberculosis. *American Review of Respiratory Diseases* **121**, 139–48.

Cross reference
Chapter 9, Complications

Case 33 A shortened leg since childhood

Presenting complaint
A 49-year-old man of Irish origin presented with a discharging sinus over the left hip.

History of presenting complaint
The sinus had been present for a few weeks. It had developed as an area of redness and discomfort, and then discharged with some relief of pain, but still continued to leak. The patient had not lost weight, and reported no systemic symptoms.

Past medical history
The patient had walked with a limp since the age of 10 years, when he had had 'an infection' in his left hip, which was treated with bed rest for 12 months, but never with drugs. The infection had resulted in his left leg becoming shortened by approximately 4 cm.

Examination
There was true shortening of the left leg, and a discharging sinus lateral to the greater trochanter.

Tests
The patient's chest X-ray was clear. The X-ray of his left hip (Fig. 33.1) showed a damaged and abnormal greater trochanter of the left femur with a little soft tissue swelling. Haemoglobin was 14.6 g/dL with an ESR of 28 mm/h.

Progress
A clinical diagnosis of tuberculous osteomyelitis was made. A biopsy was taken from the sinus, and material was sent for tuberculosis culture as well as pus from the sinus. Treatment with rifampicin, isoniazid and pyrazinamide was started. There was a reduction in the discharge from the hip sinus. After 4 weeks the patient was admitted with throat discomfort due to an acute goitre which could not be linked with his drugs or illness. The neck was explored and a normal thyroid gland was found, pushed forward by a retrothyroid abscess, from which 50 mL of pus were removed. The pus was positive for AFB on microscopy. By this time the cultures from the hip sinus were positive for mycobacteria, but the colonies were suspected of being M. bovis. This was later confirmed, with the expected resistance to pyrazinamide. The pyrazinamide was switched to ethambutol, and treatment with rifampicin/isoniazid and ethambutol was given for 2 months, followed by rifampicin/isoniazid for a further 7 months. Pus from the neck was also culture positive for M. bovis. The hip sinus healed after 2 months of revised therapy.

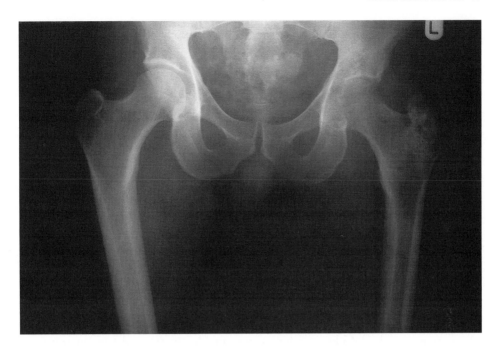

Fig. 33.1

Comment

This man had been born in the Irish Republic which, in the 1940s when he had acquired his initial infection, had a high rate of bovine tuberculosis infection. This then 'arrested' but reactivated in later life. The development of an acute retrothyroid tuberculous abscess was unexpected, and is the only case the authors have seen. M. bovis is genetically resistant to pyrazinamide, which is one of the methods by which it can be differentiated from M. tuberculosis. Clearly pyrazinamide in such cases is ineffective. Treatment should be with rifampicin and isoniazid for 9 months, supplemented by 2 months of initial ethambutol treatment. M. bovis is now uncommon in developed countries because of the effective tuberculin testing of cattle over the last 40 years which, together with pasteurization of milk, has largely eradicated the organism from both the cattle and human populations. Such cases as do occur in developed countries are now nearly all in elderly people who were infected in childhood but in whom the organism reactivates in later life. M. bovis still occurs in less developed countries.

Reference

Fanning, E.A. 1994: Mycobacterium bovis infections in animals and humans. In Davies, P.D.O. (ed.) Clinical tuberculosis. London: Chapman and Hall, 535–52.

Case 34   The man on treatment for nearly 4 years

Presenting complaint
A 31-year-old Pakistani man was seen in the clinic in January 1981 with persistent cavitation and sputum on treatment.

History of presenting complaint
The patient had been living in the UK since 1970. He had presented with cough, fever and haemoptysis in November 1976 when his chest X-ray showed right upper zone cavitation, and his sputum was smear and culture positive with fully sensitive organisms. He had been treated with rifampicin, isoniazid and ethambutol since that date, but had failed to attend on many occasions, had made return visits to Pakistan while not on therapy, and had not been supervised. He continued to have a productive cough with streak haemoptysis.

Examination
The patient weighed 45 kg and had some crackles in the right upper zone.

Tests
The chest X-ray showed persistent cavitation in the right upper zone (Fig. 34.1), Haemoglobin was 15.9 g/dL and ESR was 14 mm/h. Sputum samples were sent for microscopy and culture.

Progress
Drug treatment was stopped pending culture results and drug resistance was assumed. Sputum was negative on smear but positive on culture after 7 weeks, and the sensitivity results reported 4 weeks later showed marked resistance to rifampicin and isoniazid. The patient was then admitted to hospital for treatment, by which time sputum was smear and culture positive with the same sensitivities. In-patient treatment with ethionamide 500 mg bd, cycloserine 500 mg bd, streptomycin 0.75 g, pyrazinamide 1.5 g and ethambutol 700 mg daily was given. Monthly sputum cultures were tested, and became negative after 4 weeks of treatment. In-patient treatment was continued for 4 months, by which time the upper lobe cavity had closed. Fully supervised treatment with the remaining drugs was continued as an out-patient, again with monthly sputum cultures, with the remaining drugs for a further 7 months. All cultures were negative after the first months of treatment, and drugs were stopped 10 months after the first negative culture. The patient was followed up regularly, with cultures remaining negative. He had a spontaneous left pneumothorax treated by intercostal drain in 1985, but was discharged from follow-up with negative cultures in 1996, 14 years after stopping treatment.

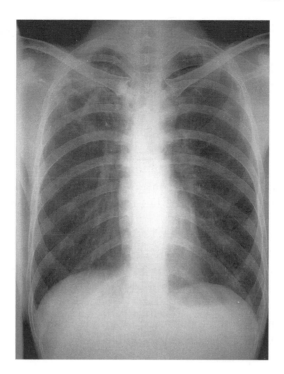

Fig. 34.1

Comment

This man developed multi-drug-resistant tuberculosis (MDR-TB) due to a combination of his non-compliance with medication and poor supervision of drug-taking and the continuance of drugs when this was clearly inappropriate. His MDR-TB was cured by scrupulous treatment as an in-patient for 4 months with five drugs, followed by fully supervised twice-daily treatment for more than 9 months after the last negative culture. Long-term follow-up confirmed clinical and bacteriological cure. Nearly all cases of MDR-TB are due to failure of treatment and management. They can be avoided by giving the correct regimen, using combination tablets to prevent deliberate or accidental monotherapy, and close monitoring of compliance either by a DOT system or by careful regular monitoring of self-medication.

Reference

Goble, M., Iseman, M., Madsen, L.A. *et al.* 1993: Treatment of 171 patients with pulmonary tuberculosis resistant to isoniazid and rifampin. *New England Journal of Medicine* **328**, 527–32.

Case 35   The lady with the destroyed lung

Presenting complaint
A 74-year-old Pakistani woman became ill while visiting relatives in a different part of the UK. Her symptoms were increased cough, streak haemoptysis and some nocturnal fever.

History of presenting complaint
The patient had had respiratory symptoms for many years, with intermittent cough and sputum. These had become worse over a 4-week period, and the development of haemoptysis caused her to seek medical attention.

Past medical history
The patient had first entered the UK in 1982 and had been found to have an abnormal chest X-ray. She was investigated and treated with rifampicin/isoniazid and ethambutol at that time, but returned to Pakistan after about 8 weeks and was treated there. She re-entered the UK in 1990, at which time her chest X-ray was again abnormal, with a destroyed left lung. Her ESR was persistently elevated at 80–100 mm/h, but repeated sputum samples were culture negative, as were *Aspergillus* precipitins.

Examination
Examination revealed signs of collapse/consolidation of the left lung.

Tests
Chest X-ray (Fig. 35.1) revealed left-sided collapse/consolidation. Sputum samples taken on admission to hospital in the other part of the UK were heavily smear positive, and treatment with rifampicin, isoniazid, pyrazinamide and ethambutol was given. The patient was discharged to her relatives, and returned to the local unit a few weeks later while on the above treatment.

Progress
Our local unit was contacted 6 weeks after the patient had commenced treatment with the report that her cultures were positive, but that sensitivity tests showed her to be highly resistant to both rifampicin and isoniazid, and initial tests also suggested some resistance to ethambutol and streptomycin as well. The patient was readmitted to an independently ventilated side-ward and was shown to be still sputum microscopy positive. Rifampicin, isoniazid and ethambutol were stopped, and treatment was changed to clarithromycin (500 mg bd), prothionamide (500 mg bd), pyrazinamide (1.5 g), ofloxacin (400 mg bd) and capreomycin (0.5 g IM daily). After 1 month the patient was microscopy negative, but she developed considerable pruritis and rash. Pyrazinamide was stopped and replaced by clofazimine (200 mg/day), with resolution of the pruritis. Repeat sensitivity tests showed high resistance to rifampicin, isoniazid

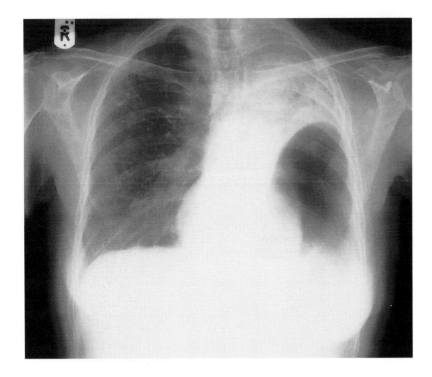

Fig. 35.1

and rifabutin but full sensitivity to ethambutol. Ethambutol (15 mg/kg) was added to the regimen. After 3 months sputum was microscopy negative, and samples from 1 month were culture negative. Capreomycin and clofazimine were stopped. Treatment continued with prothionamide, clarithromycin, ofloxacin and ethambutol. After 3 months of in-patient treatment the patient was discharged on twice daily fully supervised treatment (DOT). This was given for a further 4 months until she was admitted with bilateral peripheral gangrene due to arteriosclerosis, from which she died. The chest X-ray did not change, but monthly sputum samples remained smear and culture negative after 1 month of treatment.

Comment

This patient had a history of previous treatment which had probably been less than adequate, and which therefore substantially increased the likelihood of drug resistance. Molecular probes are now available which can give early diagnosis of rifampicin resistance on cultures and are 90 to 95 per cent accurate on microscopy-positive clinical samples. Since isolated rifampicin resistance is uncommon, any rifampicin-resistant case should be treated as for MDR-TB until proved otherwise. There needs to be full segregation of such cases in fully engineered isolation wards to prevent nosocomial transmission, particularly if other patients in the unit are immunocompromised (e.g. HIV positive). Treatment should commence with at least five drugs to which the organism is known or thought to be likely to be sensitive, and these should be continued until negative cultures are obtained. Treatment should then continue for at least a further 9 months after cultures are negative. Consideration may also have to be given to surgical resection of lung lesions under drug cover.

References

Goyal, M., Shaw, R.J., Banerjee, D.K., Coker, R.J., Robertson, B.D. and Young, D.B. 1997: Rapid detection of multidrug-resistant tuberculosis. *European Respiratory Journal* **10**, 120–24.

Iseman, M. 1993: Treatment of multidrug-resistant tuberculosis. *New England Journal of Medicine* **329**, 784–90.

Case 36 Third time lucky

Presenting complaint
A 29-year-old unmarried lady doctor, who had completed her house-officer training in the cardiology department of a hospital in Pakistan, prior to her illness, presented with a long-standing history of productive cough, fever, and haemoptysis and weight loss. Before this presentation she had already had two courses of antituberculosis treatment.

Drug history
The patient had taken rifampicin, isoniazid, streptomycin and ethambutol for 9 months when she was diagnosed as having pulmonary tuberculosis. She started to take pyrazinamide instead of streptomycin in addition to the other three drugs mentioned above when she relapsed in 1993–1994.

Family history
At the initial interview the patient was hesitant about disclosing that her younger brother had died of tuberculosis some time previously. She mentioned this later on when she was sure that the information would be kept confidential, for fear of the stigma associated with tuberculosis.

Tests
Blood count showed normocytic anaemia, and chest X-ray showed extensive cavitations occupying almost the whole of the left lung and patchy involvement of the right upper zone (Fig. 36.1).

Sputum smears were positive for AFB and a specimen was sent for AFB culture and sensitivity analysis. After 6 weeks, when the culture and sensitivity results were available, they showed resistance to rifampicin, INH, ethambutol and streptomycin, while the AFB were only sensitive to thiacetazone and pyrazinamide.

Progress
The patient was admitted to hospital and started treatment on second-line drugs which included cycloserine, ethionamide, ofloxacin, thiacetazone and isoniazid. Since cycloserine and ethionamide are not available in Pakistan, these drugs were imported at great financial cost. The patient responded well, was smear negative after 2 weeks of therapy, and remained so for over 2 years.

During treatment she was admitted to hospital on several occasions with acute exacerbations secondary to bacterial infections. At one stage she developed a huge lung abscess involving the left hemithorax which, despite conservative management, was not draining, and with the aid of the thoracic surgeons it had to be intubated. At another time the need for left-sided pneumonectomy was considered, but because of the patient's poor pulmonary function that idea had to be abandoned. After some time, in one of the follow-up visits the huge cavity

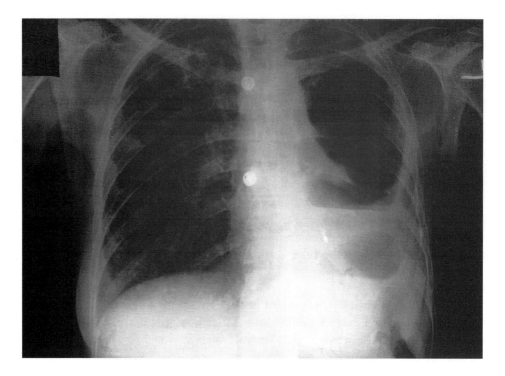

Fig. 36.1

present was seen to have collapsed, causing a shift of the mediastinum towards the left (Fig. 36.2). With perseverance and reassurance the patient completed 2 years of second-line therapy, but experienced all kinds of side-effects, including nausea, vomiting and abdominal pain, vertigo, weakness, confusion, agitation and generalized weakness. While she was in hospital her mother died of cirrhosis of the liver. Her father, who was also a doctor, died of polyarteritis nodosum soon after the patient had completed her treatment.

Comments
This patient contracted the infection from her brother, who probably died of resistant pulmonary tuberculosis. Although her compliance with first-line drugs was good, she did not respond to them, probably because she had primary resistance.

This case also illustrates various problems associated with tuberculosis. It highlights the prolonged morbidity from which the patient with tuberculosis can suffer. This young woman was first diagnosed as having tuberculosis in 1985, and she suffered from the disease until 1996, after having had two courses of first-line drugs and then second-line drugs for more than 2 years, finally being left with a destroyed lung and severely affected pulmonary functions. Not all cases have a happy ending, as the likelihood of cure in resistant pulmonary tuberculosis is

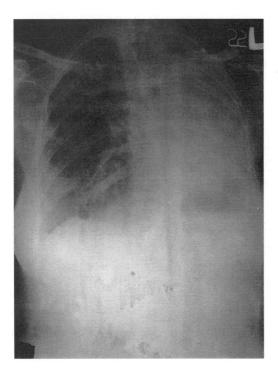

Fig. 36.2

only 50 per cent despite a response to second-line drugs. In addition, the toxic effects of the second-line drugs can make the life of such patients very wretched.

This case also highlights the social stigma and isolation that may be linked with this disease. In this case the patient was reluctant to give her family history (her younger brother dying of the disease some time previously) due to fear of isolation and stigmatization. This family is in a very precarious situation, with both parents dead and the older brother dying of tuberculosis. This patient had two sisters and a younger brother, and the prospects of them living a normal life seem fairly remote.

Case 37   The hospital doctor

Presenting complaint
A 30-year-old junior hospital doctor from India presented with cough, weight loss of 4 kg and malaise.

History of presenting complaint
The patient had been treated for tuberculosis in India 4 years previously. She had arrived in the UK approximately 3 months before the symptoms first appeared, and presented about 2 months after she first felt unwell.

Examination and tests
No specific abnormality was found on examination, apart from the presence of a persistent dry cough. Sputum was positive on direct smear for AAFB. A chest radiograph showed calcified lesions and a few scattered soft opacities in the left upper lobe (Fig. 37.1)

Outcome
A detailed history showed that the patient had been given isoniazid, rifampicin, pyrazinamide and ethambutol for tuberculosis in India. She was started on isoniazid, rifampicin, streptomycin, ethionamide and ciprofloxacin, and the

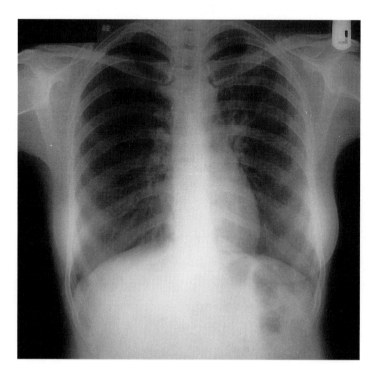

Fig. 37.1

microbiology department was contacted to request fast tracking of the specimens for culture and sensitivity. Within 1 week the patient complained of tinnitus, so the streptomycin was stopped. Four weeks after initial presentation, the sensitivity results showed resistance to streptomycin and isoniazid only. Treatment for the patient, who had been complaining of abdominal pains, probably caused by the ethionamide, was therefore changed to rifampicin, pyrazinamide, ethambutol and ciprofloxacin. Her subsequent recovery was uneventful and treatment stopped after 9 months.

Comment
This patient had relapsed after receiving four first-line drugs for tuberculosis. It was possible that she could have become resistant to all of these, but because isoniazid and rifampicin are such important drugs and the possibility of susceptibility remained, these were included in the retreatment regimen. In addition, the patient was started on three drugs that she had not taken before, namely streptomycin, ethionamide and ciprofloxacin. In retrospect the inclusion of streptomycin was a mistake, as she had presumably acquired a streptomycin-resistant strain during the first episode. Streptomycin should probably not be included in a retreatment schedule except in areas where streptomycin resistance is known to be rare. Fortunately, the patient was able to tolerate two drugs she had not received before, namely ethionamide and ciprofloxacin, until sensitivity results became available. Once it was apparent that isolates were sensitive to rifampicin and other first-line drugs, the regimen could be modified accordingly.

Contact tracing of patients and other staff was extensive, but only one other person (a 16-year-old female patient with a strongly positive tuberculin test but normal chest radiograph) was found who might have been infected by this patient. Because of known isoniazid resistance, the contact was given preventive therapy in the form of rifampicin alone for 3 months. The procedure for screening immigrant workers at occupational health services was reviewed. It was recognized by the occupational health physician that a tuberculin test performed on the patient at the time when she started work would have been positive and therefore uninformative. The occupational health physician had interviewed the patient, but in the absence of symptomatic evidence of disease a chest radiograph had not been indicated. The patient was advised to report any symptoms that might be due to tuberculosis as soon as possible, which is in fact what she did. Subsequent consultation revealed that she had not complied fully with medication during treatment for the first episode of disease.

Relapse of disease occurs in 5 to 10 per cent of patients in the UK. The extent to which this is due to lack of compliance is not known, but non-compliance must account for an appreciable proportion of such cases.

Cross reference
Chapter 1, Section 1A, Smear-positive, culture-positive disease

Case 38   The resistant brother

Presenting complaint

The 36-year-old brother of a patient known to have multi-drug-resistant tuberculosis (resistant to isoniazid, rifampicin and ethambutol) presented with a history of several months of cough and weight loss.

Progress

The patient had been a heroin abuser and admitted to smoking cannabis and tobacco regularly. A chest X-ray at presentation showed a large (3 cm) cavity in the left upper lobe and sputum was smear positive for AAFB. In view of the likely source of infection, the patient was started on isoniazid, rifampicin, pyrazinamide, prothionamide and ciprofloxacin. By the next time he attended the clinic, sensitivity results were available showing strong resistance to isoniazid and rifampicin but sensitivity to all other antituberculosis drugs. He had been unable to tolerate the prothionamide, so ethambutol was added to the regimen to give three drugs to which the patient was known to be sensitive. At the clinic 1 month later and 2 months after initial presentation his sputum smear was negative and he had put on 2 kg in weight.

Four months after presentation the patient continued to be sputum smear negative, and two of three cultures were negative.

He failed to turn up at the clinic for his next appointment, and when he did reattend he had lost 4 kg in weight and his sputum had become smear positive. He admitted to failing to take his medication, and he reluctantly agreed to have DOT. He continued on ethambutol, ciprofloxacin and pyrazinamide, and 4 months later sputum smear and culture had become negative. A sensitivity result at this time suggested resistance to ethambutol. It was decided to replace this drug with clarithromycin in order to maintain three drugs to which the organism was sensitive. The patient was unable to tolerate this or prothionamide as a third holding drug. At this time no cycloserine could be obtained, so the patient was continued on only two drugs, ciprofloxacin and pyrazinamide.

Although he maintains reasonable clinical health on this regimen and sputum remains smear and culture negative, it has been recommended that he should have a left upper lobectomy. A CT scan showed two distinct thick-walled cavities in the left upper lobe (Fig. 38.1)

Comment

This patient falls into the typical risk category for multi-drug resistance in that he is a close contact of a drug-resistant case and also a substance abuser. In terms of personality it was difficult to ensure compliance in this patient. He had refused hospital admission for more than 1 week and also refused to take intramuscular medication. The approach of starting him on isoniazid and rifampicin plus at least three drugs to which he was likely to be sensitive was followed. Unfortunately, adverse effects, the development of ethambutol

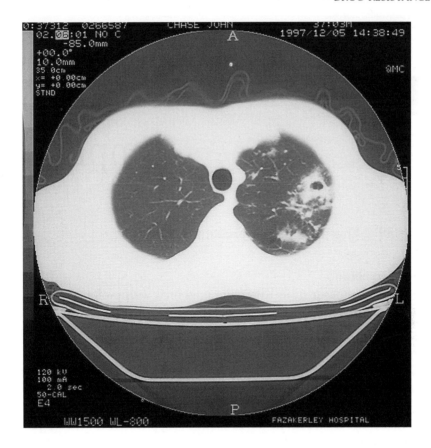

Fig. 38.1

resistance and the temporary unavailability of cycloserine mean that he is only able to take two weak drugs to which the bacteria are sensitive.

As the disease was apparently confined to a single lobe on CT scanning (Fig. 38.1), this patient was a good candidate for surgical intervention. One year after surgery, he remains smear and culture negative, and continues on three second-line drugs.

Reference
Iseman, M.D., Madsen, L., Goble, M. and Pomerantz, M. 1990: Surgical intervention in treatment of pulmonary disease caused by drug-resistant M. *tuberculosis. American Review of Respiratory Diseases* **141**, 623–5.

Cross reference
Chapter 1, Section 1A, Smear-positive, culture-positive disease

5

Poor compliance

Case 39 The Sudanese merchant

Presenting complaint
A 35-year-old businessman in Khartoum presented with prolonged cough, fever and weight loss.

History of presenting complaint
The patient first developed symptoms which consisted of feeling tired, cough, fever and weight loss. After 6 weeks he presented to his nearest chest clinic, where he was diagnosed as having tuberculosis. He was prescribed treatment with isoniazid and thiacetazone for 12 months, supplemented with streptomycin daily for the first 2 months. He took his treatment irregularly but had improved after 8 months, at which time he stopped his treatment altogether. Several months later he presented again with similar symptoms. Because he was a merchant and had sufficient financial resources, he travelled to Saudi Arabia where he consulted a specialist. He was told he again had tuberculosis, and was prescribed a combination of medications, most probably including rifampicin, to be taken for 6 months on a daily basis. After 4 months on these medications he saw no further need for them. His symptoms returned once again, and he returned to the chest clinic, where he was now given five medications, namely isoniazid, rifampicin and ethambutol for 8 months supplemented with strepto- mycin for 2 months and pyrazinamide for 2 months. Seven years later, he was seen again at the clinic, having attended on numerous occasions previously. On this occasion, he was tired, had lost weight and had a chronic, persistent cough with intermittent haemoptysis.

Examination
Physical examination showed a wasted man with a temperature of 39°C. No lymph nodes were palpable. There were crepitations in both upper zones of the chest.

Tests

Sputum smears were positive for AFB. Cultures grew M. *tuberculosis* which, on susceptibility testing, was found to be resistant to isoniazid, streptomycin and rifampicin, the only medications for which susceptibility testing had been carried out. Chest radiograph showed extensive infiltration and cavitation, greater in the apices, but present bilaterally and throughout the lung fields. The chest films were subsequently lost and were unavailable for review.

Outcome

The patient was given isoniazid to take continuously, and was instructed to take precautions (when coughing to cover the mouth and nose, and to avoid contact with young children). His condition improved, but he was never free of symptoms.

Comment

This patient represents a case of multi-drug-resistant tuberculosis that was essentially incurable in the circumstances of limited resources characteristic of most low-income countries. Although reserve drugs might be obtained, they are very expensive (over $US 2000 for the medications alone), must be administered over a very long period of time (18–24 months) and have quite an unsatisfactory outcome. Such patients may live for years and with the potential to infect all those around them.

Case 40   The unhappy divorcee

Presenting complaint
A 20-year-old Nepali woman presented because she had experienced cough and haemoptysis for 6 months.

History of presenting complaint
The patient lived in a remote hill region of Nepal where she was married to a farmer and had one small child. When she first began to cough she was afraid to attend the clinic, but when she started to cough blood, she finally presented for examination.

Past medical history
The patient had been healthy prior to this illness, and had no known contact with tuberculosis.

Examination
Physical examination showed a pale, thin woman with a temperature of 39.5°C. There were crepitations in the right upper chest, but examination was otherwise normal.

Test
Sputum was examined and shown to be positive for AFB.

Outcome
The patient was informed that she had tuberculosis and was asked to attend the clinic daily for treatment with isoniazid, rifampicin, pyrazinamide and ethambutol, to be continued for 2 months, to be followed by isoniazid and ethambutol to be taken at home daily for 6 months. After 3 weeks of treatment, her husband expelled her from their home because of the stigma of tuberculosis, and then took another wife. The patient's family would not allow her to live with them because of her illness, so she became a homeless beggar.

Comment
This young woman represents a story that is all too common, particularly in the Middle East and in the Indian subcontinent. The stigma attached to tuberculosis is still so great, particularly among women, that diagnosis is frequently delayed, and indeed some individuals prefer to die at home without ever presenting to the health service. If an unmarried woman is known to have tuberculosis, she will never marry. Moreover, no respectable family would agree to marry any of their members to such a family.

The management of tuberculosis in such a setting also differs from that usually practised in industrialized countries. Patients are requested to attend daily for DOT during the period when they are taking rifampicin. Furthermore, there are no chest radiograph and no culture facilities available nearby. Such cases are treated with a standardized protocol which gives treatment results equivalent to those in any industrialized country. The usual management consists of daily thiazina (thiacetazone and isoniazid) after the initial intensive phase, which provides the most effective means of preventing rifampicin resistance. However, some locations, such as Nepal, elect not to use this treatment and put themselves at risk of compromising ethambutol and, subsequently, rifampicin.

Case 41   Returning from the Diaspora

Background
Filipinos represent the largest expatriate population in the world. In 1987 it was estimated that there are over 3 million Filipino overseas contact-workers (OCWs), mostly working in the Middle East and aboard ships. Indeed, some people have referred to this as the second Diaspora. With increasing ease of cross-country travel in a shrinking global village it is important for disease and treatment guidelines to take into consideration the growing threat of Diaspora diseases.

Presenting complaint
A 43-year-old Filipino who for the past 7 months had been working as a plumber in Saudi Arabia returned home because of dyspnoea and cough.

History of presenting complaint
Two months previously the patient had experienced low-grade afternoon fevers, recurrent cough productive of yellowish phlegm, anorexia and mild weight loss while working in Saudi Arabia. He consulted a company physician who prescribed cough preparations. These produced slight relief of his symptoms but the low-grade fever persisted. The patient continued to work.

One month later he consulted again and was admitted to hospital and given antituberculosis therapy. Smear was reported to be positive (++) although sputum AFB culture was negative. A chest X-ray taken at that time showed infiltration of the right upper and middle lung field. The patient was told he had pulmonary tuberculosis (PTB) and diabetes. He was given insulin (20 units/day) and was kept in isolation for 2 weeks, during which time there was a slight improvement in his condition. He was discharged afebrile. A few days after discharge, his cough worsened and was associated with pleuritic chest pain. He was subsequently repatriated back to the Philippines where he consulted a private physician who prescribed medication that gave no relief. He then presented at the university hospital and admission was advised.

Examination
Physical examination showed a moderately built, ambulatory man, afebrile and not in any form of respiratory distress, who was not tachycardic but was tachypnoeic (respiratory rate = 28 breaths/min). There were diminished breath sounds over the right upper lung field and absent breath sounds over the right base.

Tests
Initial chest X-ray showed complete collapse of the right lung with air-fluid consistent with hydropneumothorax. The patient subsequently underwent tube thoracostomy which drained 1 L of orange-yellow slightly turbid fluid

consistent with empyema thoracis. Pleural fluid showed a WBC of 2916 mm^3 (predominant polymorphonucleocytes) and protein concentration of 24.6 g/dL. Pleural fluid Gram stain as well as bacterial cultures were negative, and AFB smear and culture using Lowenstein'–Jensen medium were also negative.

Outcome

The patient was started on empirical treatment consisting of Rifater (HRZ) (4 tablets once daily), Cefdinir (300 mg/day) and Ciprofloxacin (250 mg BID) and insulin injections. Repeat X-ray showed re-expansion of the right lung with persistent soft infiltrates in the right middle to lower lung field. The patient was subsequently discharged after 5 days of confinement. He had one out-patient follow-up.

The patient was readmitted exactly 1 month later (Christmas Day 1996) because of dyspnoea and pus that was spontaneously draining from the former thoracostomy site which had previously healed. A repeat X-ray was performed which showed recurrence of pneumohydrothorax with pleural thickening, although there were still some lung markings in the right upper field. The patient subsequently underwent another tube thoracotomy and turbid pleural fluid was again drained. There was strong persistent bubbling from the water-sealed bottle, and the patient was subsequently diagnosed as having broncho-pleural fistula. Because of the persistent collapse, a second posterior tube was subsequently inserted, the two tubes were then hooked to a three-way suction system and there was a re-expansion of the right lung on the seventh day of hospitalization. Pleural fluid WBC showed a packed field, the Gram stain was again negative for AFB smears, and cultures were negative. Medications given included Rifater, and streptomycin was added with clarithromycin (500 mg/day) and clindamycin (300 mg QID). The initial blood sugar concentration was 252 mg/dL. The patient was referred to a diabetologist who administered humulin (30 units/day), and the blood sugar level was eventually controlled. On the ninth day of hospitalization the patient asked the thoracic surgeon to convert the two tubes to modified Heimlich valves, and he was discharged after 2 days. Subsequent out-patient follow-up of the pleural fluid showed Gram-negative bacilli (+1) with light growth of Pseudomonas aeroginosa.

One month later the patient was again admitted because of loss of consciousness due to elevated blood sugar (492 mg/dL), but stayed for only 3 days. He continued with the Heimlich valves, which were attached to a sterile plastic pouch that was replaced daily. After 3 days his blood sugar concentration dropped to 169 mg/dL after humulin injections, 42 U/day. He was discharged on treatment with Rifater, streptomycin, clarithromycin and cefuroxine (1500 mg/day). Four days after discharge the tubes were removed. The patient was subsequently located in his home town in connection with this case report and is currently doing well (off insulin), has gained weight and is essentially asymptomatic almost 1 year after the above events. He is due to return for follow-up.

Comment

Diseases of Diaspora have been described as illnesses attributable to mass migration and international travel. The obviously very complicated case described above is a classic example of this. It also depicts the plight of overseas workers in search of better opportunities and income when their families are transported to strange lands and become increasingly susceptible to diseases such as tuberculosis, despite stringent screening procedures. This phenomenon presents a challenge to clinicians world-wide, highlighting the need for tuberculosis doctors to reassess treatment guidelines when these are applied to migrant workers.

Case 42   The defaulter

Presenting complaint
A 26-year-old man presented with a 4-week history of cough and with weight loss and reduced appetite.

History of presenting complaint
The patient had a history of pulmonary tuberculosis 6 years previously. At the time he received antituberculosis treatment from a general practitioner for 3 months, after which time he failed to attend. He consulted another general practitioner 5 years later when he experienced some cough and weight loss. A chest X-ray taken during that visit showed infiltration shadows in both upper zones as well as a cavitating shadow in the left upper zone. Antituberculosis treatment was restarted, but the patient again failed to attend after receiving treatment for only 2 months. The exact nature of the drugs received by the patient was not known for either episode, nor was the sputum status at the time of diagnosis known.

The patient attended the chest clinic 7 months later, presenting with a 4-week history of cough, weight loss and reduced appetite. He had not received any medication for his symptoms prior to his visit to the chest clinic.

Past medical history
There was no past medical history of relevance.

Examination
Physical examination showed a thin young man in a satisfactory general condition. He was afebrile. No glands were palpable, and examination of the chest, cardiovascular system, gastrointestinal and central nervous system did not reveal any abnormalities.

Tests
A chest radiograph showed the same infiltrative shadows in both upper zones, and a cavitating shadow in the left upper zone, as were observed in the private film taken 9 months earlier. There was also some deterioration in the left lower zone. Blood tests, including a complete blood profile, liver and renal function tests were normal. Sputum examination was positive for AFB by smear.

Outcome
The patient was put on supervised treatment with five drugs, streptomycin, isoniazid, rifampicin, pyrazinamide and ethambutol, at the chest clinic. The importance of adherence to the prescribed treatment was emphasized. The patient responded clinically to supervised treatment at the chest clinic, and his sputum became negative after 2 months. The drug regimen was changed to isoniazid, rifampicin and ethambutol at 3 months when culture and sensitivity

test results became available, and revealed M. *tuberculosis* sensitive to first-line drugs. The patient continued to receive supervised treatment at the chest clinic for a further 6 months. A chest X-ray taken on the day of completion of treatment showed improvement in both the upper zone shadows, with closing down of the left upper zone cavity.

Comment

Patient non-compliance has been identified as the most important determinant of the outcome of tuberculosis treatment. It is also a major obstacle to the elimination of the disease. The consequences of non-compliance include treatment failure, relapse, additional treatment, additional expense, increase in drug resistance, and death.

Tuberculosis can be cured and prevented in virtually all cases if patients follow a prescribed treatment regimen for an adequate period of time. Directly observed treatment, short course (DOTS), has been emphasized by the World Health Organization as the most important strategy in tuberculosis control programmes. DOTS refers to the process whereby a health-care worker or trained lay person watches while a patient swallows antituberculosis drugs over the 6–9-month treatment period. The drugs can be administered in daily or intermittent regimens in a wide range of clinical settings or at home, work, school or any convenient designated area. The importance of DOTS is exemplified by the above case, in which the patient had a relapse following previous episodes of unsupervised treatment by general practitioners. Clinical, bacteriological and radiological improvements were observed after a 9-month period of fully supervised treatment at the chest clinic.

DOTS has been used successfully in many countries, where it has resulted in a reduction in the overall rates of tuberculosis, primary and acquired resistance, as well as relapse. It has also been shown to be one of the most cost-effective measures in medical intervention.

Extrapulmonary disease

6

Case 43   A febrile immigrant with an effusion

Presenting complaint
An 18-year-old Pakistani woman presented with fever, dry cough and breathlessness which had persisted for 2 weeks.

History of presenting complaint
The patient had been in the UK for 12 months. She had experienced fever and 'flu-like' symptoms for 2 weeks, with weight loss of 7 kg. She had also had a dry non-productive cough and had developed breathlessness on moderate effort. There was no past history of note.

Examination
The patient was toxic, with a temperature of 39.0°C and signs of a large right pleural effusion (Fig. 43.1).

Tests
Haemoglobin was 10.0 g/dL normochromic and ESR was 123 mm/h. Serum proteins showed an albumen level of 29 g/L and a globulin level of 37 g/L. The tuberculin test was strongly positive. Pleural aspiration, biopsy and drainage were performed. The fluid showed an exudate (protein 51 g/L), which was heavily lymphocytic on cytology. Pleural biopsy showed multiple necrotic granulomata with palisaded epithelioid histiocytes and lymphocytes. Pleural fluid was later culture positive at 6 weeks for M. *tuberculosis* fully sensitive to first-line drugs.

Progress
A total of 4 L of fluid were drained, and treatment commenced on the basis of the lymphocytic exudate. Treatment was started with rifampicin, isoniazid and

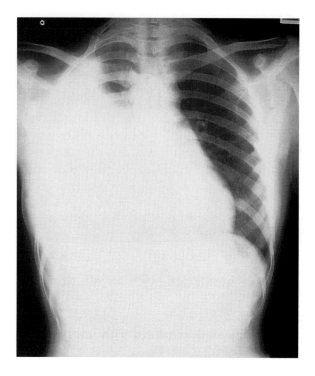

Fig. 43.1

pyrazinamide orally. The patient remained toxic and was vomiting despite normal transaminases. Treatment with IV rifampicin and isoniazid, together with streptomycin and hydrocortisone, was given for 4 days. This stopped the vomiting and reduced the fever. Treatment was then switched back to oral rifampicin, isoniazid and pyrazinamide with prednisolone (30 mg/day). Treatment with steroids was gradually withdrawn over 2 months. Pyrazinamide was stopped when full sensitivity was confirmed, and treatment was continued with rifampicin/isoniazid as combination tablets for a total of 6 months. At the end of treatment the chest X-ray showed only a minimal basal pleural reaction, and the ESR was 4 mm/h.

Comment

The immediate working diagnosis here was tuberculosis. Any person in an ethnic minority group and with a pleural effusion, particularly if a recent immigrant, should be regarded as having tuberculosis until proved otherwise. Treatment was commenced on the basis of a lymphocytic exudate and a positive tuberculin test. Pleural fluid is positive on culture in up to 50 per cent of cases, but is rarely microscopy positive, and usually takes 4 to 6 weeks to yield a positive culture. Similarly, pleural biopsy is not positive in all cases due to the patchy distribution of granulomata. The biopsy is more likely to be positive if multiple samples are taken, the operator is experienced, or the biopsy is under direct vision (e.g. at thoracoscopy). Standard short-course chemotherapy is appropriate for pleural disease. Corticosteroids may be needed in addition for systemic effects, and there are some data to support more rapid clearance of fluid with corticosteroids. Large pleural effusions need to be drained, while smaller amounts can be aspirated or left to resolve on medication. Continued fluid production or the need for repeated fluid aspirations is an indication for corticosteroids. In low-income countries treatment based on clinical findings and a positive tuberculin test may be appropriate. In HIV-coinfected patients there is an increase in pleural disease, but the tuberculin test is more likely to be negative.

References

Lee, C.H., Wang, W.J., Lan, R.S. *et al.* 1988: Corticosteroids in the treatment of tuberculous pleurisy. A double blind, placebo controlled, randomised study. *Chest* **94**, 1256–9.

Ormerod, L.P., McCarthy, O.R., Rudd, R.M. and Horsfield, N. 1995: Short-course chemotherapy for tuberculous pleural effusions and culture negative tuberculosis. *Tubercle and Lung Disease* **76**, 25–7.

Case 44   A breathless old lady

Presenting complaint
A 69-year-old white woman was seen with malaise and a pleural effusion.

History of presenting complaint
The patient had had flu-like symptoms 4 months earlier and had then been admitted to hospital 8 weeks earlier with right pleuritic pain and fever. She had been treated for pneumonia and showed clinical improvement, but 50 mL of blood-stained fluid had been aspirated at that time. She had been a non-smoker for over 20 years, but she had had some exposure to industrial asbestos 45 years earlier. Persistent pleural shadowing was seen on the chest X-ray, and the patient was referred to the chest clinic.

Past medical history
Appendicectomy and cholecystectomy were the only features of the history.

Examination
The patient's weight was 65 kg with signs of a small right pleural effusion.

Tests
Chest X-ray (Fig. 44.1) showed right basal shadowing which was mainly pleural. Haemoglobin was 12.1 g/dL and ESR was 37 mm/h. The pleural fluid that was removed several weeks earlier had shown no malignant cells, and had a protein content of 46 g/L. Liver function and biochemical profile were normal.

Progress
A CT of the thorax was arranged, but within a few days the pleural fluid aspirated earlier was reported to be culture positive for AFB, later confirmed as M. *tuberculosis* that was fully sensitive to all drugs. The CT was cancelled, and treatment with Rifater was started. The patient now recalled that a cousin had died of tuberculosis 22 years earlier. Her treatment was uneventful until week 8 when vomiting and jaundice developed. Treatment was stopped with an ALT concentration of 3690 IU/L. There had been considerable improvement in the chest X-ray. Liver function had returned to normal after 3 weeks, so rifampicin/isoniazid were restarted, but the ALT concentration decreased to 165 IU/L and bilirubin rose to 32 mmol/L within 10 days. The drugs were again stopped. Liver function returned to normal within 5 days, ethambutol (15 mg/kg) was started and isoniazid was re-introduced, initially at 50 mg/day for 3 days and then at 300 mg/day, with liver function remaining normal. Treatment with isoniazid and ethambutol was continued for a further 7 months. The chest X-ray showed only minimal blunting of the right costophrenic angle on completion of treatment.

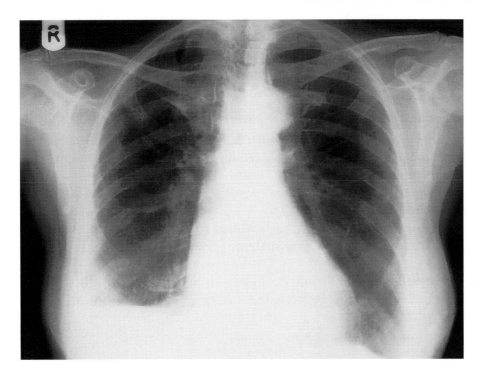

Fig. 44.1

Comment

Tuberculosis was not suspected in this older white woman, and secondary malignancy or mesothelioma was considered more likely. However, pleural fluid had been sent for culture despite the small probability of infection. Pleural tuberculosis usually gives a straw-coloured lymphocyte-rich exudate, but the effusion can be heavily blood-stained. Pleural biopsy might have given the diagnosis, but may only yield granulomata in 50 per cent of cases, multiple biopsies being more likely to give a positive result. Tuberculous pleural effusion is usually an immediate post-primary phenomenon, but can occur as a reactivation phenomenon in older age.

Reference

Mungall, I.P.F., Cowen, P.N., Cooke, N.T. et al. 1980: Multiple pleural biopsy with the Abrams needle. Thorax 35, 600–2.

Cross reference

Chapter 2, Management of adverse drug reactions

Case 45   A case of empyema

Presenting complaint
A 38-year-old Pakistani man was seen with a 5-day history of fever.

History of presenting complaint
The patient had returned 1 week earlier from a 7-week visit to Pakistan, and the fever had developed 2 days after his return. He had lost 4 kg in weight over a 6-month period.

Past medical history
The patient was a non-smoker but admitted to drinking 90 units of alcohol a week until 3 months before presentation.

Examination
The patient was febrile at between 38.5 and 39.0°C, and showed signs of a right pleural effusion.

Tests
Haemoglobin was 11.7 g/dL normochromic and the white cell count was 6.1×10^6/mL. Bilirubin was normal but ALT at 56 IU/L (normal range < 45 IU/L) and alkaline phosphatase at 161 IU/L (normal range < 145 IU/L) were slightly elevated. Chest X-ray (Fig. 45.1) showed a right pleural effusion with some widening of the upper mediastinum. Aspiration of the pleural effusion showed 400 mL of purulent fluid, which was sent for culture.

Progress
Because of the purulent fluid the patient was treated as an empyema case, with intravenous cefotaxime, gentamycin and metronidazole. A right basal chest drain was inserted and a further 800 mL of purulent fluid were drained. His fever did not respond to 7 days of the above antibiotics. The pleural fluid showed predominantly lymphocytes on cytology, was negative on standard and anaerobic cultures, and was an exudate (protein 55 mg/L). The pleural fluid was negative on direct microscopy for AFB. A trial of antituberculosis treatment with Rifater 5 tablets (for weight 63 kg) was given, and the fever responded within 7 days. The drain was removed and the patient began to regain weight. His dose of Rifater was increased to 6 tablets when he reached 65 kg in weight. After 5 weeks positive cultures were received for M. tuberculosis, later shown to be fully sensitive. Liver function monitoring because of the patient's history of abnormal liver function tests and previous excessive alcohol consumption showed improvement to normal over 4 weeks. The pyrazinamide was stopped when full sensitivity was confirmed. He was treated with a further 4 months of rifampicin/isoniazid and weighed 76 kg on completion of treatment. There was some

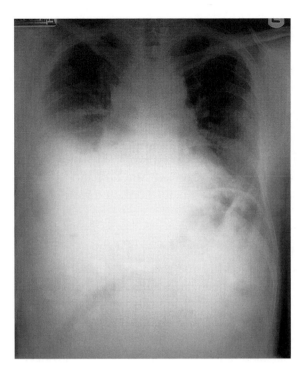

Fig. 45.1

residual pleural scarring, and the patient's spirometry showed a mild restrictive defect (FEV_1 2.35/2.75 L, compared to predicted value of 3.40/4.21 L).

Comment

In view of the short history and purulent pleural fluid, a non-tuberculous empyema was first suspected. The lack of response to broad-spectrum antibiotics, and particularly the finding of a lymphocytosis in the purulent fluid, rather than a polymorph leucocytosis, suggested tuberculosis. Pleural fluid was negative on microscopy, but was later culture positive. Tuberculous empyemas may be microscopy positive, whereas this is very rarely the case for 'standard' tuberculous pleural effusions. Indeed, culture confirmation may only be obtained in 50–60 per cent of effusions. A tuberculous empyema should be managed in the same way as any other empyema, with appropriate antibiotics, drainage of pus, and consideration of decortication. It is possible in this case that the lung function at the end of treatment might have been better if a decortication had been performed, but the patient was reluctant to consider surgery.

Case 46   The obese barman

Presenting complaint
A 47-year-old barman presented with a 3-month history of breathlessness.

History of presenting complaint
The patient, who worked part time in a social club bar, complained that for 3 months he had experienced progressive breathlessness. He had a persistent smoker's cough which had not changed, and he had lost no weight. There was no significant past history. The patient drank in excess of 50 units of alcohol a week.

Examination and tests
The patient was obese (105 kg) and there was clinical evidence of a right-sided pleural effusion. He had a low-grade fluctuating pyrexia. The presence of an effusion was confirmed on chest X-ray (Fig. 46.1). One litre of straw-coloured fluid, which was an exudate, was aspirated from the chest. This fluid was negative on direct smear for AAFB, but a pleural biopsy performed at the same time showed a few granulomata. A Mantoux test was strongly positive (25-mm induration to 10 tuberculin units).

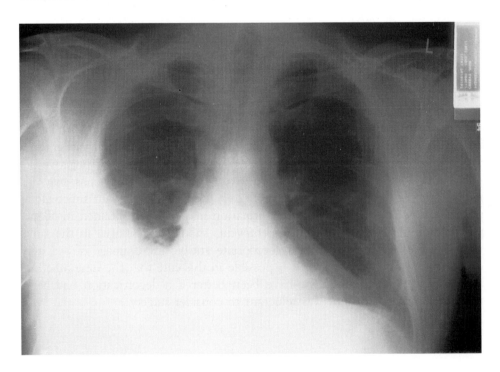

Fig. 46.1

Outcome

The patient was started on triple antituberculous chemotherapy. Initially there was no apparent response. The pyrexia continued and he showed no symptomatic improvement. After 1 week of continuing high temperature he was started on oral prednisolone (60 mg). Within 24 h his temperature had returned to normal and he felt considerably better. He was discharged from hospital and continued on steroids in addition to full antituberculous chemotherapy for 4 months. The effusion had resolved by the end of the third month of treatment. Antituberculous drugs were continued for 6 months.

Comment

Pleural effusions are usually associated with primary tuberculosis, and are caused by hypersensitivity reactions to tubercles on the pleura. Bacilli in the fluid are sparse, so the smear is usually negative. Negative culture is also not uncommon. Rarely they may become heavily contaminated with bacilli and a tuberculous empyema may result. Diagnosis is usually made by histology and culture of the pleura itself. If pleural fluid can be removed, then a pleural biopsy can and should be performed. Standard chemotherapy for 6 months is sufficient, and steroids are reported to speed the resorption of fluid, although recent evidence suggests that they make no difference to the final outcome.

This patient had continuing pyrexia despite several days of treatment. The fact that this was immediately suppressed by steroids suggests a hypersensitivity phenomenon, although whether this was due to the initial pathology or to the antituberculous chemotherapy is unclear. Steroids have an important role in suppressing the hypersensitivity reaction of tuberculosis itself or of the drugs used in treatment, and should be considered if pyrexia persists beyond 1 week of treatment in the presence of a firm diagnosis of tuberculosis.

The absence of weight loss or of any symptoms other than those caused by the effusion itself suggests a primary disease in this patient. Pleural effusion in the elderly is more likely to be due to reactivation of a primary infection, so-called post-primary disease, and weight loss and other symptomatology are usual.

Reference

Rossi, G.A., Balbi, B. and Manca, F. 1987: Tuberculous pleural effusions. *American Review of Respiratory Diseases* **138**, 575–9.

SECTION 6B MEDIASTINAL LYMPHADENOPATHY

Case 47 An asymptomatic contact

Presenting complaint

An 18-year-old asymptomatic household contact was seen for tuberculosis screening.

History of presenting complaint

The patient was seen as a contact of his younger brother, who had been found to have tuberculous mediastinal glands on new-immigrant screening. He had been born in the UK, had had neonatal BCG vaccination, but had then spent 9 years in Pakistan, returning 8 years before his screening. There was no past medical history of note.

Examination

Other than a positive tuberculin skin reaction there were no findings. No peripheral lymphadenopathy was found.

Tests

The tuberculin test was strongly positive (Heaf grade 4). Chest X-ray showed minimal widening of the mediastinum. Routine blood tests were normal.

Progress

Repeat chest X-ray after 3 months (Fig. 47.1) showed definite paratracheal widening. This was presumed to be tuberculosis on clinical grounds, because the family screening had also found that the patient's father had sputum-smear-positive tuberculosis. Triple therapy (isoniazid, rifampicin and pyrazinamide) was commenced, ethambutol was not given because the father's organisms were fully sensitive. Initial compliance was less than ideal in that the patient missed a few days of treatment and ran out of drugs. Close supervision was introduced with random urine tests and visits. His clinical progress was uneventful, with resolution of the mediastinal lymphadenopathy within 3 months, the X-ray being normal at the end of standard short-course chemotherapy. The X-ray was also normal 4 years later when the same patient was seen as a contact of a different case.

Comment

Mediastinal lymphadenopathy accompanied by a strongly positive tuberculin test in ethnic minority groups should be regarded as tuberculosis until proved otherwise. In this case there were two other family members with clinical disease. However, no symptoms were present, and only X-ray screening showed disease. Routine mediastinoscopy for tissue and culture is not necessary in such

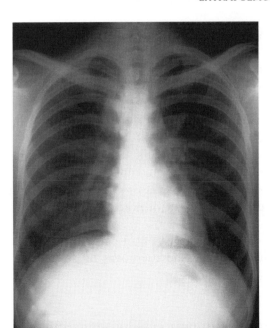

Fig. 47.1

cases, but should be reserved for those cases where there are clinical doubts or there is failure to improve with correctly taken chemotherapy.

Reference
Farrow, P.R., Jones. D.A., Stanley. P.J. *et al.* 1985: Thoracic lymphadenopathy in Asian residents in the UK: role of mediastinoscopy in initial diagnosis. *Thorax* **40**, 121–4.

Case 48   Another recent immigrant

Presenting complaint
A 28-year-old recent Indian immigrant was seen with chest pain and streak haemoptysis.

History of presenting complaint
The patient had been living in the UK for 1 year. For 1 month he had had a cough with streaks of blood, and he complained of dull retrosternal discomfort over the same period. He had no fever or sweats, and no significant weight loss. There was no past medical history of note.

Examination
There were no clinical signs, and there was no fever, peripheral lymphadenopathy or hepatosplenomegaly.

Tests
Chest X-ray showed right paratracheal lymphadenopathy (Fig. 48.1). Haemoglobin was 14.2 g/dL, ESR was 14 mm/h, and biochemistry and liver function were normal. Tuberculin tests were negative. Two sputum samples were sent for AFB microscopy, which was negative.

Progress
It had been expected that the tuberculin test would be strongly positive and that treatment for tuberculosis would be started. A CT of the thorax was arranged, which confirmed right paratracheal lymphadenopathy with enhancement of the periphery of the gland and a non-enhancing lower density centre, both features being very suggestive of tuberculous lymphadenopathy (Fig. 48.2). The tuberculin test was still negative on repeat testing, so the patient was referred for mediastinoscopy.

Prior to mediastinoscopy the surgeon performed rigid bronchoscopy when a nodular lesion in the lateral wall of the right intermediate bronchus was found. This was biopsied and bled profusely, so mediastinoscopy was not performed. Histology showed dense inflammation with many epithelioid granulomata and scattered multinucleate giant cells of Langhan's type consistent with tuberculosis. Treatment with four drugs (rifampicin, isoniazid, pyrazinamide, ethambutol) was commenced and was uneventful. The lymphadenopathy resolved over 3 months. Sputum cultures before and after bronchoscopy were negative on culture for AFB. Pyrazinamide and ethambutol were stopped after 2 months, and treatment was completed with rifampicin/isoniazid for 4 months.

Comment
Tuberculous mediastinal glands were strongly suspected clinically, but the tuberculin tests were negative. The CT scan features were also highly suggestive

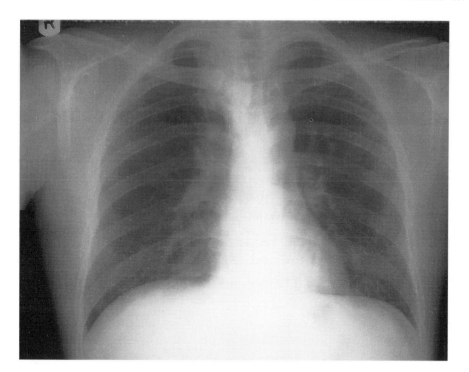

Fig. 48.1

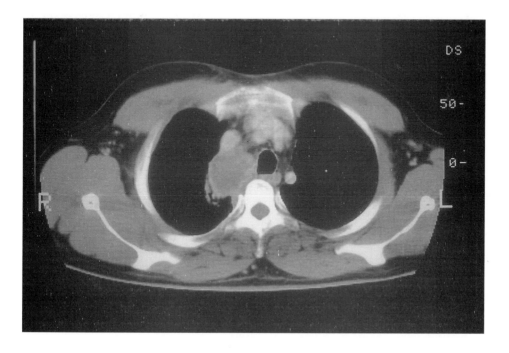

Fig. 48.2

of tuberculosis, with ring-enhancing nodes with a hypodense centre. Mediastino-scopy was considered because of the negative tuberculin tests. Rigid broncho-scopy showed unexpected endobronchial disease and gave a histological diagnosis. Fibre-optic bronchoscopy would have given the same information, and might have allowed washing for cultures. Fibre-optic bronchoscopy does have a yield of positive cultures from washings in mediastinal lymphadenopathy when there is no visible endobronchial disease, and also shows unexpected endobronchial disease in some cases.

References

Chang, S., Lee, P. and Perng, R. 1988: Clinical role of bronchoscopy in adults with intrathoracic tuberculous lymphadenopathy. *Chest* **93**, 314–17.

Im, J.G., Itoh, H. and Shim, Y.S. *et al.* 1993: Pulmonary tuberculosis: CT findings – early active disease and sequential change with antituberculosis treatment. *Radiology* **186**, 653–60.

Case 49   The man with the worsening X-ray

Presenting complaint
A 25-year-old Indian man presented with malaise, fatigue and weight loss.

History of presenting complaint
The patient was born in the UK and had last visited India 2 years before presentation. He had experienced malaise for 4 months with fatigue but no cough, and intermittent daily headaches over the same period. He had also lost 3.5 kg in weight. There was no past history of note and no family history of tuberculosis.

Tests
Examination was normal. Haemoglobin was 13.3 g/dL, WCC was 4.7×10^6/mL, the lymphocyte count was 0.9×10^6/mL and ESR was 22 mm/h. Globulin was 45 g/L. The tuberculin test was strongly positive (Heaf 4). Chest X-ray showed early infiltration in the left upper zone.

Progress
A clinical/radiological diagnosis of tuberculosis was made and treatment with Rifater started (for body weight 70 kg). This was tolerated without problems, but after 8 weeks the chest X-ray had worsened (Fig. 49.1), showing definite mediastinal glands and left basal pleural shadowing. A rub was heard over the left base. CT of the thorax showed enlarged right paratracheal glands, a small left basal effusion and multiple irregular densities peripherally in the apices of both lungs. Pleural aspiration attempts were unsuccessful. The CD4 count was 290 μL (normal range 450–1050 μL). HIV testing was negative. Because of concerns about the possibility of drug resistance or other diagnosis, bronchoscopy and mediastinoscopy were performed. Bronchoscopy was normal. At mediastinoscopy a hard paratracheal gland was found which gushed pus on biopsy. The pus was positive for AFB on microscopy, and histology showed multiple caseating granulomata. Ethambutol (15 mg/kg) and clarithromycin (500 mg bd) to cover the possibility of drug resistance were added to the patient's antituberculosis drugs, and prednisolone (25 mg/day) because of the pleural reaction and development of lymphadenopathy. Treatment was fully supervised, and after 8 weeks there was a substantial improvement in both the pleural shadowing and the mediastinal glands. Cultures from the mediastinoscopy were negative for M. tuberculosis. One month later clarithromycin and pyrazinamide were stopped and steroids were tailed off. Treatment was continued with rifampicin, isoniazid and ethambutol for a further 5 months. The patient gained a further 5 kg in weight and his CD4 count returned to normal.

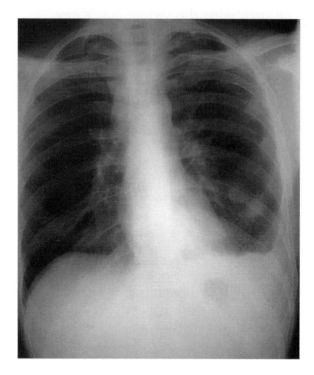

Fig. 49.1

Comment

The deterioration after 8 weeks of treatment raised a number of questions. Was this due to non-compliance, although random urine tests had been positive for rifampicin? Paradoxical enlargement of glands is recognized in the treatment of lymph-node tuberculosis (either peripheral or mediastinal), but there had been no apparent nodes on the initial chest X-ray, and this phenomenon is less common with pyrazinamide-containing regimens. Was there a non-tuberculous pathology or copathology? The lymphopenia and raised globulins together with a moderately reduced CD4 count could have been due to more disseminated tuberculosis but HIV co-infection needed to be excluded. After exclusion of HIV and histological confirmation of tuberculosis, two drugs were added, pending culture results, to cover the possibility of drug resistance (a single drug should never be added to a regimen that is possibly failing). Further treatment was fully supervised, even though non-compliance had not been confirmed. Because no sensitivities were available, because of negative cultures, ethambutol was given together with rifampicin and isoniazid to cover the possibility of undetected isoniazid resistance.

Reference
Swanson Beck, J., Potts, R.C., Kardjito, T. and Grange, J.M. 1985: T4 lymphopenia in patients with active tuberculosis. *Clinical and Experimental Immunology* **60**, 49–54.

Case 50   The hot Indian

Presenting complaint
A 45-year-old Indian man presented with 2 months of sweating and malaise.

History of presenting complaint
The patient had emigrated from Northern India to the UK approximately 20 years previously. For 2 months he had noticed that he was having frequent episodes of sweating. These would last a few hours at a time. Initially they occurred only at night, but latterly they had occurred at any time and he had started to feel generally unwell and had lost some weight. He had no specific symptoms relevant to the chest, in particular no cough or breathlessness.

Past medical history
There was no past medical history of relevance, and no known contact with tuberculosis.

Examination
Physical examination showed a thin but generally well Indian man. His temperature was 38.5°C. No glands were palpable and no abnormality was detected in the chest, cardiovascular, gastrointestinal or central nervous system.

Tests
A plain chest X-ray was normal. ESR was 80 mm/h, haemoglobin was 12.9 g/dL, and WCC was 6.9×19^6/mL. Urea and electrolytes were normal, but the liver function test was mildly deranged with gamma-glutamyl transferase (GGT) 56 IU/L (normal range 20–40 IU/L) and alkaline phosphatase 125 U/L (normal range 50–110 U/L). A full screen for pyrexia of unknown origin (PUO) was performed, including screening for parasites and ova, but there were no abnormal findings. During these investigations the patient continued to have a temperature of up to 38.5°C on most days. A CT scan of the chest showed enlarged mediastinal glands which had not been apparent on plain chest X-ray. Mediastinoscopy and biopsy were performed which showed a generalized inflammatory reaction and numerous AFB on direct staining (Plates 50.1 and 50.2). Specimens subsequently grew M. tuberculosis which was fully sensitive to first-line drugs.

Outcome
The patient was started on quadruple therapy consisting of isoniazid, rifampicin, pyrazinamide and ethambutol, because infection might have been acquired in India where drug resistance is prevalent. He made a reasonable recovery and his high temperature resolved. Five months after treatment had started his chest X-ray showed marked widening of the mediastinum, and a CT of the chest

confirmed enlargement of the mediastinal glands. A second operation was performed to remove as much of the matted enlarged glands as possible. Specimens from biopsies at the second operation remained sterile on culture. The patient is continuing on quadruple therapy, and high-dose oral steroids have been added.

Comment

Unusual presentations of tuberculosis in immigrants from the Indian sub-continent to the UK are well documented. Not only do they have a much higher incidence of disease than the white population, but also the site of disease is much more frequently extrapulmonary. Histology often shows the absence of granuloma formation, presumably due to reduced immunity of uncertain aetiology. The pattern of disease in these individuals has been compared with HIV-positive tuberculosis, which also results in much higher rates of extrapulmonary disease. The phenomenon has been termed 'acquired immunodeficiency of immigration', and may result from impairment of macro-phage function as a result of a marked reduction in vitamin D on immigration. This patient presented as a case of pyrexia of unknown origin with mediastinal lymphadenopathy due to tuberculosis. The diagnosis was only made by mediastinal gland biopsy, when specimens were taken for histology and culture.

Patients usually respond satisfactorily to conventional treatment, but in some individuals lymphadenopathy may increase despite adequate treatment. The management of this situation is contentious. Surgical intervention may be required as a debulking procedure, but it is likely that fistulae will result, which may be slow to heal, and further glandular enlargement may occur. Steroid treatment may have a role, but there are no reliable trial data to support this approach.

Reference

Davies, P.D.O. 1998: Tuberculosis and migration. In Davies, P.D.O. (ed.), *Clinical Tuberculosis*, 2nd edn. London: Chapman & Hall, pp. 365–82.

SECTION 6C PERICARDIAL DISEASE

Case 51 The man with right upper quadrant pain

Presenting complaint
A 26-year-old Pakistani man presented with right upper quadrant abdominal pain.

History of presenting complaint
The patient had been in the UK for 4 years with no return visits to Pakistan. He had had a feeling of epigastric fullness for 5 months, but this had become more severe over a period of 4 days and had spread to the right upper quadrant. For 1 week he had felt breathless when lying flat. There was no past medical history of note.

Examination
The surgical examination showed some right upper quadrant tenderness, and three finger-breadths of enlarged liver.

Tests
Abdominal X-ray was unhelpful. Ultrasound showed normal spleen and kidneys. The liver was slightly enlarged with increased vascularity, and a small amount of right pleural fluid was present. The sodium level was 119 mmol/L and other electrolytes were normal.

Progress
Because of the presence of pleural fluid on ultrasound, a chest X-ray was performed (Figs 51.1 and 51.2) which showed marked cardiomegaly. Examination by a physician showed the jugular venous pressure (JVP) to rise with inspiration (Kussmauhl's sign), but no pulsus paradoxus. An echocardiogram (Fig. 51.3) showed a large pericardial effusion. An echoguided sub-xiphisternal aspiration was performed and 600 mL of thick blood-stained fluid were removed. This showed red blood cells and predominantly lymphocytes on cytology, and had a protein content of 68 g/L. AFB were not seen on microscopy. A diagnosis of tuberculosis pericarditis was made and treatment was commenced with triple therapy and prednisolone (60 mg/day). Weekly echocardiography showed rapid resolution of fluid with approximately 100 mL detectable after 1 week and minimal fluid by week 2. Steroids were then reduced to 50 mg/day for 3 weeks and subsequently to 40 mg/day. The patient's symptoms largely disappeared in the first week. Culture from the pericardial fluid was positive for M. *tuberculosis* at 5 weeks, and full sensitivities were confirmed by 8 weeks. Pyrazinamide was then stopped and prednisolone was reduced to 30 mg/day and withdrawn at a rate of 10 mg every 2 weeks. Antituberculosis therapy was stopped after 6

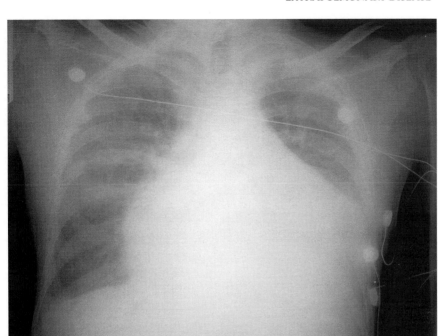

Fig. 51.1

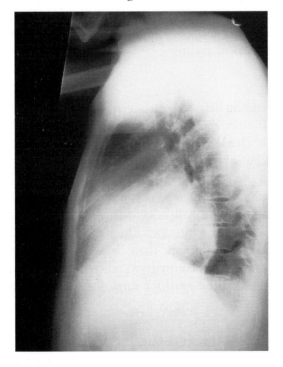

Fig. 51.2

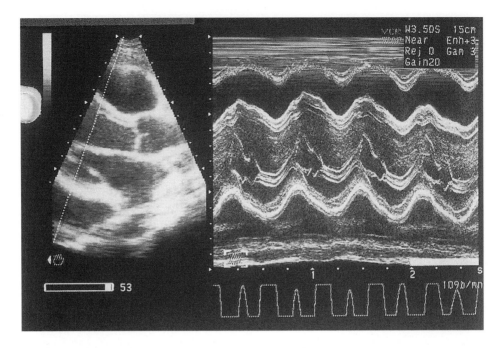

Fig. 51.3

months. Chest X-ray on completion of treatment was normal (cardiothoracic ratio (CTR) 12.5/27). Yearly echocardiograms for the last 3 years have shown no evidence of constriction or recurrence.

Comment

The symptoms presenting here were believed to be those of hepatic congestion, but breathlessness is often the dominant symptom. Ascites and leg oedema can also be present. The chest X-ray was highly suggestive of pericardial fluid, and this was confirmed by echocardiogram.

Pericardiocentesis was performed under ultrasound control, but can be performed without ultrasound in areas of the world with few resources. A clinical diagnosis was made from the lymphocyte-rich exudate. Prednisolone (60 mg/day) was given in addition to antituberculosis drugs because clinical trials have shown that, in pericardial effusion, there is a much reduced death rate and progression to constriction. In constrictive tuberculosis pericarditis steroids also reduce the death rate and the need for surgical pericardectomy.

Reference

Strang, J.I.G., Kakaza, H.H.S., Gibson, D.G. *et al.* 1988: Controlled trial of complete open drainage and prednisolone in the treatment of tuberculous pericardial effusion in Transkei. *Lancet* ii, 759–63.

Case 52 A case of pyrexia of unknown origin, with developments

Presenting complaint
A 27-year-old Pakistani man presented with fever, malaise and headache.

History of presenting complaint
The patient had lived in the UK for 7 years, and had been unwell for 3 weeks, with intermittent fever, weight loss of 8 kg and mild headache. There was no past history of note.

Examination
The patient was febrile at 38.7°C, but there were no focal findings.

Tests
Initial chest X-ray was normal. Haemoglobin was 12.7 g/dL normochromic with an ESR of 75 mm/h. Biochemical profile, collagen screen and abdominal ultrasound were normal, and lumbar puncture was also normal. The tuberculin test was positive (Heaf 3). Fever up to 39.0°C continued.

Progress
A trial of antituberculosis treatment was commenced with rifampicin, isoniazid and pyrazinamide. The fever began to settle and the patient was allowed to go home. A few days later he was readmitted with a recurrence of fever, anorexia and vomiting. Liver function was normal. The antituberculous drugs were stopped for 48 h and the vomiting settled. Repeat abdominal ultrasound was normal, but repeat chest X-ray (Fig. 52.1) showed an enlarged heart shadow and a right pleural effusion. Pleural aspiration showed a lymphocyte-rich exudate, but was later culture negative. Echocardiogram showed a pericardial effusion of 100–150 mL, and there was no evidence of tamponade. Pericardiocentesis was not performed. Treatment with rifampicin (600 mg) and ethambutol (900 mg) was restarted without problems. After the echocardiogram, isoniazid (300 mg) and prednisolone (60 mg) daily were also added. The fever settled rapidly, and the pericardial effusion resolved over 4 weeks on serial echocardiogram monitoring. Treatment totalling 9 months of rifampicin and isoniazid, supplemented by 2 months of initial therapy with ethambutol, was given, with the prednisolone being progressively withdrawn over 3 months. At the end of treatment the chest X-ray was normal, the ESR was 6 mm/h the patient had gained 13 kg.

Comment
When this patient presented the picture was really one of a pyrexia of unknown origin. There was no initial clinical or X-ray evidence of pericardial involvement. This became apparent 2 weeks into the illness, when there was also

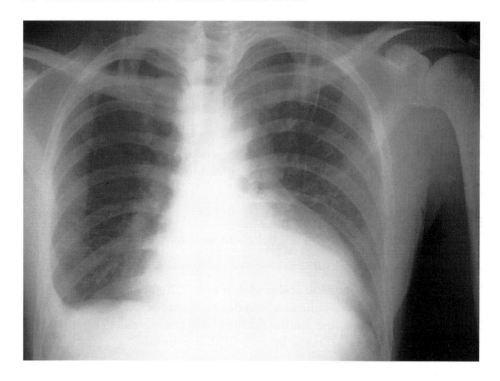

Fig. 52.1

evidence of a pleural effusion. The vomiting was attributed to pyrazinamide, without evidence of hepatitis. The pericardial effusion was not causing haemodynamic embarrassment, and was considered to be too small to tap safely. In this case the pleural and pericardial involvements were felt to have developed against the background of 'cryptic miliary' or disseminated tuberculosis. A 6-month short course of chemotherapy would have been adequate with a pyrazinamide-containing regimen in the absence of central nervous system involvement, but a 9-month regimen was needed because pyrazinamide was omitted.

Reference
Strang, J.I.G., Kakaza, H.H.S., Gibson, D.G. *et al.* 1987: Controlled trial of prednisolone as an adjuvant in treatment of TB constrictive pericarditis in Transkei. *Lancet* **ii**: 418–22.

Cross references
Chapter 2, Management of adverse drug reactions; Chapter 6, Section 6G, Miliary disease

SECTION 6D   BONE AND JOINT

Case 53   Lower back pain

Presenting complaint
A 30-year-old Pakistani woman presented with low back pain which was getting worse.

History of presenting complaint
The low back pain had been present for 6 months, having initially been intermittent, but it had become persistent, and was requiring regular analgesia. Movement of the lower back in all directions was reduced, but there was no pain in the legs, nor were there neurological symptoms. In addition, the patient had felt generally unwell for 1 month, with malaise and a few episodes of fever. She had no past history of note, and had been living in the UK for 5 years.

Examination
There was some loss of lumbar lordosis, with reduced spinal movements in all directions at lumbar level, with tenderness on percussion but no gibbus or long-tract neurological signs.

Tests
ESR was 66 mm/h, globulin was 43 g/L and the tuberculin test was strongly positive (Heaf 3). Plain X-ray (Figs 53.1 and 53.2) showed an L3/4 discitis with substantial destruction of the body of L4.

CT scan showed similar features, and there was an associated inflammatory mass but no abscess to aspirate. There was no encroachment on the spinal canal. Chest X-ray was normal. The patient's weight was 56 kg.

Progress
A clinical diagnosis was made of tuberculosis of the spine. There was no indication for immediate surgical intervention, and no pus to aspirate para-spinally. Treatment with Rifater (5 tablets/day) was given, with analgesia and an NSAID for symptoms. The patient's symptoms slowly improved. Pyrazinamide was stopped after 2 months, and rifampicin/isoniazid were given for a further 4 months, treatment being ambulant throughout. Bony fusion occurred by 4 months, and was confirmed by CT scan, with the thin remnant of L4 fusing to L3 without spinal canal encroachment. Management throughout was by joint medical/orthopaedic assessment. ESR fell to 17 mm/h and the patient's weight had increased to 62.8 kg by the end of treatment.

Comment
In this case there had been substantial bone destruction at presentation, but this together with a discitis formed the clinical diagnosis. The discitis is usually at a

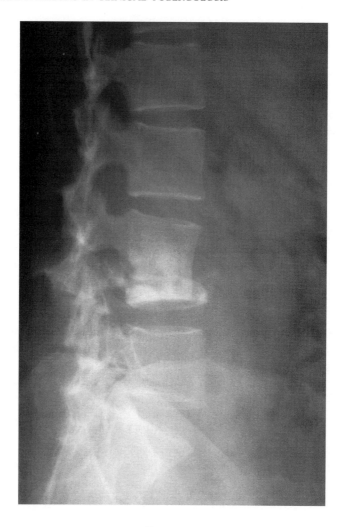

Fig. 53.1

single level, but multiple levels which are not necessarily contiguous may be involved. Isotope bone scan may show increased uptake before there are plain X-ray changes. If there are any long-tract neurological signs or symptoms, or sphincter involvement, then orthopaedic or neurosurgical assessment is mandatory to determine whether decompression is required. Nuclear magnetic resonance (NMR) scanning is very helpful in assessing possible spinal cord compression. Spinal cord compression can occur from an extradural abscess or from bony collapse and encroachment into the spinal canal. Most cases of bone/joint disease have a normal chest X-ray, but this can be part of a disseminated process (as in Case 54) or with respiratory disease (as in Case 57).

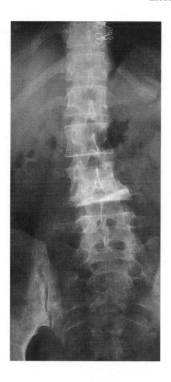

Fig. 53.2

References
Bell, G.R., Stearns, K.L., Bomietti, P.M. and Boumphrey, F.R. 1990: MRI diagnosis of tuberculous vertebral osteomyelitis. *Spine* **15**, 462–5.

Hodgson, S.P. and Ormerod, L.P. 1990: Ten-year experience of bone and joint tuberculosis in Blackburn 1978–87. *Journal of the Royal College of Surgeons of Edinburgh* **35**, 259–62.

Case 54 Right-sided abdominal pain and malaise

Presenting complaint
A 59-year-old Asian woman was seen with right-sided abdominal pain of some months' duration.

History of presenting complaint
The pain had been present for 5 months, was described as of a burning nature, and more recently had been radiating round from the back. The pain was unrelated to eating. It was possibly precipitated by movements such as bending or turning. The patient had been investigated by a general surgeon with no abnormality found on abdominal examination, blood tests or abdominal ultrasound. During the previous 2 weeks she had experienced a few fevers and mild headache but no photophobia. She had been referred for an orthopaedic opinion.

Past medical history
The patient had lived in the UK for 20 years with no serious illnesses.

Examination
The patient was febrile at 39°C. There were no abdominal findings, but minor spinal tenderness was present on percussion over the upper lumbar spine, and rotation to the right reproduced the symptoms to some extent.

Tests
The plain X-rays (Fig. 54.1) showed early erosive changes in the L1/2 disc space with some narrowing of the disc space suggestive of a discitis. The orthopaedic surgeon suspected tuberculosis and performed a chest X-ray (Fig. 54.2) which showed widespread granularity suggestive of miliary disease. He brought the X-rays to the chest clinic with the patient, who was admitted. Isotope bone scan showed marked uptake in T12/L1 and L1/2 disc spaces. Because of fever and mild headache a lumbar puncture was performed which showed a protein concentration of 3.34 g/L, a glucose level of 1.8 mmol/L and WBC of 46×10^6 cells/mL with 95 per cent monocytosis. Gram and Ziehl-Nielsen (ZN) stains were negative, and ESR was 32 mm/h.

Progress
As well as cerebrospinal fluid (CSF), early morning urine and sputum samples were sent for AFB culture. Treatment with triple therapy was commenced, but ethambutol was omitted because of reduced visual acuity due to cataracts. The fever settled over 10 days, but a repeat lumbar puncture after 10 days showed a protein concentration of 5.5 g/L, a glucose level of 1.4 mmol/L and WBC of 95×10^6 cells/mL. CT brain scan showed no evidence of tuberculomas or hydrocephalus. Prednisolone (50 mg daily) was added to the patient's treatment.

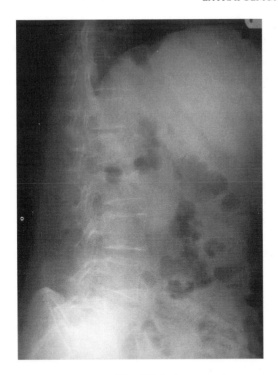

Fig. 54.1

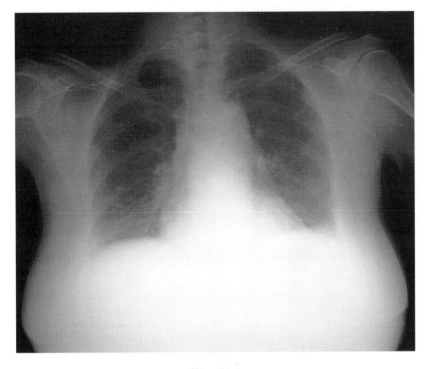

Fig. 54.2

After a further 2 weeks, CSF showed significant improvement. After 6 weeks cultures from sputum, CSF and urine were positive, and the organism was fully sensitive. Pyrazinamide was stopped after 2 months. The chest X-ray had cleared by 3 months, but rifampicin and isoniazid were continued for a total of 12 months because of the involvement of the central nervous system. The pain in the right side of the abdomen improved as bony healing occurred, but the patient needed occasional analgesics.

Comment

The pain was thought to be referred pain from nerve root irritation in the disc spaces, and diagnosis was delayed because of the lack of direct local symptoms. The changes on the plain X-rays were subtle, but because of an awareness of the 80–fold increased rate of bony tuberculosis in ethnic-minority patients, the orthopaedic surgeon took a chest X-ray in view of the patient's recent fever. The diagnosis of miliary tuberculosis, of which the tuberculous spinal discitis was a part, was rapidly established. The isotope bone scan shows more than plain X-rays, and may be positive before there are X-ray changes.

Reference

Humphries, M.J., Sister Gabriel, M. and Lee, Y.K. 1986: Spinal tuberculosis presenting as abdominal symptoms – a report of 2 cases. *Tubercle* **67**, 303–7.

Case 55   Pain in the leg and a limp

Presenting complaint
A 20-year-old Indian woman was seen with pain in the left leg and a limp.

History of presenting complaint
Although the patient had only arrived in the UK 6 weeks earlier, she had experienced back pain for 9 months and pain radiating down the left leg for 4 weeks. The pain in the left leg was worse on weight bearing, and she had developed a limp. She had also become aware of discomfort and swelling in the left groin.

Past medical history
The patient had no history of medical illnesses, but her father had had tuberculosis 5 years earlier.

Examination
The patient was very thin at 36 kg, had a 5-cm swelling in the left groin and 30° fixed flexion of the left hip due to psoas spasm. There were no neurological signs.

Tests
Chest X-ray was normal. Haemoglobin was 9.6 g/dL, with an MCV of 73.5 fL and an ESR of 88 mm/h. CT scan of the lumbar spine (Fig. 55.1) showed destruction of the L4 vertebra with large (left greater than right) psoas abscesses.

Progress
In total 20 mL of pus were aspirated from the swelling in the left groin, which was positive on microscopy for AFB and subsequently positive on culture for M. tuberculosis, which was fully sensitive. Surgical drainage of the abscesses was performed from an anterior approach with 1.0 L of pus being removed from the left and 500 mL being removed from the right. Treatment with rifampicin, isoniazid and pyrazinamide was commenced. Some fullness and fluctuation continued in the left groin, and 50 mL of fluid were removed at 6 weeks. Pyrazinamide was stopped at 2 months when sensitivities were available. Repeat CT scan showed no collections but did reveal psoas oedema. Prednisolone commencing at 30 mg/day was given, reducing over 2 months. At the end of 6 months of treatment the patient had gained 9 kg in weight, and the spine X-ray showed some L4/5 disc space reduction, but she now had full hip movement and pain-free 90° straight leg-raising with no groin swelling. She remained well during the 12-month follow-up.

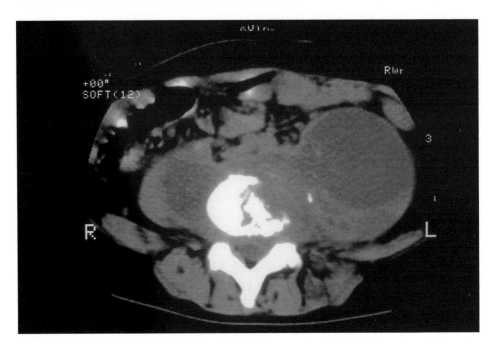

Fig. 55.1

Comment

Tuberculosis of the spine may present with what is essentially a cold abscess causing symptoms. This can be extradural, causing spinal cord compression and requiring surgical drainage, sometimes with stabilization. The more common presentations are either psoas abscesses which pass down the psoas sheath and point below the inguinal ligament, or more lateral paraspinal abscesses which discharge alongside the spine or in the loin. In the cervical spine, cold abscesses can occasionally cause dysphagia with posterior pharyngeal compression. Aspiration of pus together with the underlying X-ray changes usually confirm the diagnosis. The abscesses can discharge, and a sinus occurs in up to 15 per cent of cases. There may need to be formal surgical drainage, as in this case, but healing of the sinus must be from the base, and takes between 2 and 4 months depending on size and depth.

Case 56   A painful wrist

Presenting complaint
A 62-year-old Indian woman was seen with a 2-month history of a painful right wrist.

History of presenting complaint
During the preceding 2 months the patient had developed progressive discomfort in the right wrist, initially on movement and then all the time. Some swelling and slight redness had become apparent after 4 weeks. There was limitation of movement in both extension and flexion.

Past medical history
There was no past medical history of note.

Examination
There was swelling and slight redness of the right wrist, which also spread on to the dorsum of the hand. There was no other joint swelling and general examination was normal.

Tests
Haemoglobin was 13.2 g/dL normochromic with an ESR of 56 mm/h. Biochemistry was normal. Chest X-ray was normal, and X-ray of the right wrist showed bone erosion of the head of the third metacarpal (Fig. 56.1).

Progress
A diagnosis of tuberculous osteomyelitis was suspected. The lesion was explored under general anaesthetic, and material from the damaged area was sent for histology and mycobacterial culture. Treatment with rifampicin, isoniazid, pyrazinamide and ethambutol was commenced pending results. The histology confirmed tuberculosis with caseating granulomas and Langhans' giant cells, with scanty AFB visible on ZN staining. Cultures from the biopsy material were positive for M. tuberculosis at 6 weeks. The swelling in the wrist and dorsum of the hand improved substantially over 2 months, with the biopsy scar healing rapidly. When full sensitivity of the organism was confirmed, pyrazinamide and ethambutol were stopped. Treatment was completed with rifampicin/isoniazid for a further 4 months. The final result was excellent, with virtually normal movement of the wrist and no deformity.

Comment
Any monoarthritis in an individual from an ethnic-minority group should be considered to be tuberculosis until proven otherwise. The site of such monoarthritis can literally be any joint, but the hip, knee and elbow are the commonest sites. Tuberculous arthritis does occur in white patients, but is much

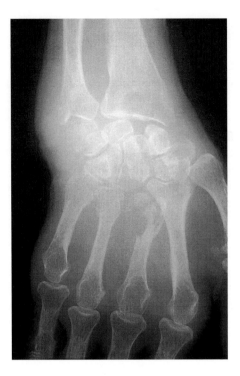

Fig. 56.1

less common, and there is often a long delay between the onset of symptoms and the diagnosis, unless biopsy and appropriate cultures for mycobacteria are taken. Six-month short-course chemotherapy should be used for bone and joint tuberculosis. The drug therapy should be undertaken by a physician who is experienced in the treatment of tuberculosis, but the mechanical aspects of the case should be dealt with by the orthopaedic surgeon, the two doctors working as a collaborative team.

Case 57   The case of the swollen finger

Presenting complaint
A 21-year-old Asian woman was seen with swelling of the left third finger that had persisted for 4 months.

History of presenting complaint
The patient had arrived in the UK from Pakistan 6 years earlier, and had made no return visits and had no past medical history of note. The third finger of her left hand had started to swell over a period of 4 months, with no history of trauma. There had been no constitutional symptoms or weight loss.

Examination
There was diffuse swelling of the digit but with sparing of the tip. Movement of the metacarpophalangeal (MCP) and proximal interphalangeal (PIP) joint was restricted by the swelling. There was little erythema.

Tests
X-ray showed minimal osteoporosis of the third proximal phalanx and some soft-tissue swelling of the digit, but no bone erosion. Blood tests and an isotope bone scan were performed, pending the results of which the patient was given flucloxacillin. The ESR was 70 mm/h with a globulin concentration of 46 g/L and an alkaline phosphatase activity of 364 IU/L. An aspiration from the soft tissue of the finger yielded no pus or fluid.

Progress
The isotope bone scan (Fig. 57.1) showed increased uptake in both the ulna shafts, the left third metacarpal, and the right third and fourth meta-carpophalangeal joints. Plain X-rays showed a lytic lesion in the left ulna. A chest X-ray (Fig. 57.2) showed bilateral mediastinal lymphadenopathy. The digit had not changed on flucloxacillin treatment. Aspiration now yielded 0.5 mL of pus from the soft tissues. Treatment with quadruple therapy (isoniazid, rifampicin, pyrazinamide and ethambutol) (15 mg/kg) was commenced. After 4 weeks, M. tuberculosis was grown from the pus and was confirmed to be fully sensitive to all first-line drugs. The digit returned to normal size over a period of 2 months. Ethambutol and pyrazinamide were then stopped, and treatment was completed with rifampicin/isoniazid for a further 4 months. The lymphadenopathy resolved over the course of treatment and the blood tests returned to normal.

Comment
In this case bone and joint disease presented with soft-tissue swelling and without constitutional symptoms. The majority of cases of bone and joint disease have normal chest X-rays, although the original site of infection is pulmonary. A

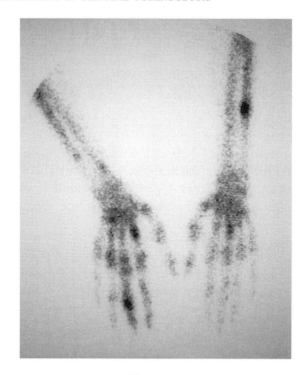

Fig. 57.1

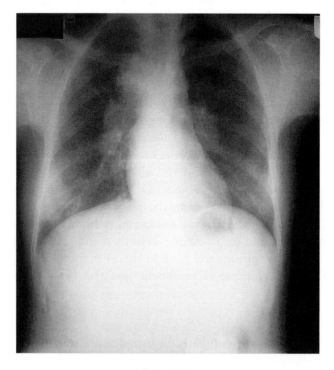

Fig. 57.2

minority of cases have evidence of past or current tuberculosis which aids in the diagnosis of the bone and joint infection. Bone and joint disease can occur at multiple sites even in non-immunocompromised patients (in this case six sites), and can occasionally simulate metastatic disease. Six months of short-course chemotherapy are satisfactory for bone and joint disease.

Reference
Ormerod, L.P., Grundy, M. and Rahman, M.A. 1989: Multiple tuberculous bone lesions simulating metastatic disease. *Tubercle* **70**, 305–7.

Case 58   The chronically restricted shoulder

Presenting complaint
A 28-year-old white manual worker was seen with limitation in movement of his right shoulder.

History of presenting complaint
Restriction in movement of the shoulder had been present since a sporting injury 10 years earlier. This was now interfering with the patient's manual job and had gradually worsened.

Past medical history
There was no past medical history of note.

Examination
There was considerable restriction of movement of the right shoulder in all directions, particularly in abduction. There were no other abnormalities.

Tests
The X-ray showed a minor erosive lesion above the greater tuberosity of the humerus (Figs 58.1 and 58.2). Arthroscopy was performed, during which

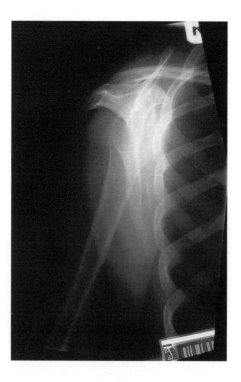

Fig. 58.1

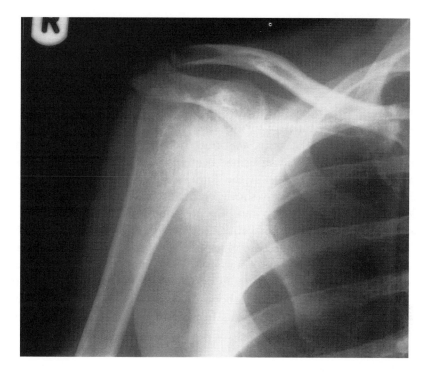

Fig. 58.2

numerous small loose fibrous bodies were found and removed, and a large rotator cuff injury was also found. The patient was referred to an orthopaedic surgeon with an interest in the shoulder region, who arranged an NMR scan of the shoulder. This showed a gross arthropathy with a markedly increased soft-tissue signal, suggesting a chronic indolent infection, and tuberculosis was queried.

Progress

A second arthroscopy was performed approximately 4 months after the first one. The entire humeral head was found to have been destroyed, and the joint space was filled with a substance described as 'sand'. This was washed out and samples were sent for histology (which showed only necrotic bone with no granulomata) and culture. Standard cultures were sterile, but M. tuberculosis was grown after 5 weeks. The humeral X-rays also showed a calcified area in the right upper zone of the lung. Treatment with triple therapy was commenced and initially went well, but at 2 months a posterior discharging sinus developed at the shoulder. The organism was fully sensitive and regular compliance monitoring had been satisfactory. The sinus was explored and debrided, and material was sent for AFB culture which was subsequently shown to be negative. Triple therapy was continued until negative cultures were received (3 months after commencement of treatment), when pyrazinamide was stopped and prednisolone (40 mg daily) was added to the rifampicin/isoniazid. The sinus was dressed regularly and it gradually healed, with the steroids being tailed off over a 3-month period. Although the infection was cured, the patient was left with a major limitation of the shoulder, and arthrodesis is being considered.

Comment

Because of the relative rarity of tuberculosis in a young white man, with a total incidence of 2 in 100 000, this was not thought to be likely. Initially the orthopaedic concern was that sepsis had been introduced at the first arthroscopy. The finding of M. *tuberculosis* in the joint, and the evidence on X-ray of a calcified scar in the lung, clearly showed that this was not the case. A sinus, or scrofuloderma, developed which can be a presentation or complication of bone and joint tuberculosis in 15 per cent of cases. After drug resistance and poor compliance had been excluded, debridement was performed. After confirming negative cultures, the corticosteroids were added because the aggressive immune response to tuberculosis can sometimes contribute to such sinus development. When there has been considerable bone destruction there can be significant residual mechanical/mobility problems from joint damage that require ortho-paedic treatment for improvement.

References

Davies, P.D.O., Humphries, M.J., Byfield, S.B. *et al.* 1984: Bone and joint tuberculosis in a national survey. *Journal of Bone and Joint Surgery* **66B**, 326–30.

Yates, V.M. and Ormerod, L.P. 1997: Cutaneous tuberculosis in Blackburn district (UK): a 15-year prospective series, 1981–95. *British Journal of Dermatology* **136**, 483–9.

SECTION 6E   ABSCESSES

Case 59   Marked weight loss and a few abscesses

Presenting complaint
A 24-year-old South African Asian presented with weight loss of over 10 kg and fever.

History of presenting complaint
The patient had lived in South Africa since birth and had only been in the UK for the last 2 years. The weight loss had occurred over 2 months with fever and mild epigastric pain. There was no past history of note, and there were no respiratory symptoms.

Examination
The patient was febrile at 38.9°C, with a swelling over the right sternoclavicular joint and a small discharging abscess in the skin above the right groin. There was a healed abscess over the anterior sternum, and there was no lymphadenopathy or hepatosplenomegaly.

Tests
Haemoglobin was 9.6 g/dL normochromic, and the white cell count was 6.4×10^6/mL with 21 per cent lymphocytes. Globulin was elevated at 44 g/L, but liver function and albumen were normal. The tuberculin test was completely negative. The CD4 count was reduced at 0.39×10^6/mL, but HIV testing was negative. Chest X-ray and abdominal ultrasound were normal.

Progress
The patient continued to be febrile up to 39°C and to lose weight down to 46 kg. Biopsies and cultures were taken from the skin abscess near the groin and from the swelling over the sternoclavicular joint. The latter was found to be due to necrotic bone from the medial head of the clavicle. Antituberculous quadruple therapy (isoniazid, rifampicin, pyrazinamide and ethambutol) was commenced pending the results. The fever responded within 7 days, and histology showed granulomata in both biopsies. Treatment was continued and positive cultures were obtained from both lesions after 4 weeks. By 2 months there had been a weight gain of 11.2 kg and healing of both abscesses. Sensitivity testing showed sensitivity to rifampicin/ethambutol and pyrazinamide, but the isoniazid result had to be repeated for technical reasons. Full therapy was continued pending the results of the repeat isoniazid test, which confirmed full sensitivity. Pyrazinamide and ethambutol were then stopped and treatment with rifampicin/isoniazid was continued for a total of 6 months. The patient's weight gain totalled 19.2 kg over the 6-month treatment period.

Comment

Disseminated or extensive tuberculosis can lead to a negative tuberculin response initially. HIV infection was excluded as a cause of this tuberculin negativity, but the CD4 count was moderately depressed. This can occur in disseminated tuberculosis and may explain the tuberculin anergy, but it improves as a response to treatment takes place, in this case returning to normal in 2 months. A trial of treatment pending results is often indicated if no immediate diagnosis is reached. As there was no clinical or investigation evidence of CNS involvement, a 6-month short-course treatment was given, the initial phase being prolonged until full sensitivity was confirmed.

Reference

Onwbalili, J.K., Edwards, A.J. and Palmer, L. 1987: T4 lymphopenia in human tuberculosis. *Tubercle* **68**, 195–200.

Case 60   A swelling in the thigh

Presenting complaint
A 42-year-old Pakistani woman was seen with a swelling in the left posterior thigh.

History of presenting complaint
The patient had arrived from Pakistan in 1991 with no return visits. She had been aware of a swelling in the left posterior thigh for a few months, and there was little pain, but she had had intermittent fever and some undefined weight loss. There was no other past medical history of note.

Examination
A deep swelling was palpable in the hamstring muscles, with a full range of movement of both the knee and the hip. There was no overlying erythema.

Tests
Plain X-rays showed no bony abnormality. ESR was 34 mm/h and globulin was raised at 45 g/L. A CT scan was performed (Fig. 60.1) which confirmed a collection of fluid deep in the muscles. This was aspirated under local anaesthetic, with standard culture and AFB microscopy being negative. Chest X-ray showed a calcified primary complex on the right.

Progress
This complex was considered by the orthopaedic surgeon to be likely to be a tuberculous cold abscess, and the patient was referred to the chest service. Treatment was commenced with Rifater and ethambutol (15 mg/kg). A few weeks later, cultures from the original aspiration were reported to be positive for *M. tuberculosis* which was highly resistant to isoniazid but fully sensitive to other first-line drugs. Rifater was stopped and treatment with rifampicin 450 mg, ethambutol 700 mg and pyrazinamide 1.5 g daily (for weight 45 kg) was given for

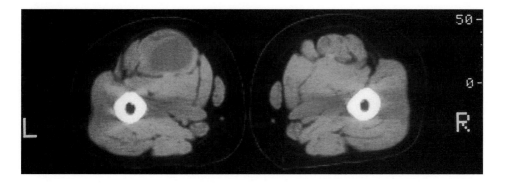

Fig. 60.1

2 months. The swelling resolved during this period. Pyrazinamide was then stopped and rifampicin and ethambutol were continued for a further 7 months. The patient's weight increased from 45 kg to 53 kg during this time and the dosage of rifampicin was increased to 600 mg and that of ethambutol to 800 mg when she reached 50 kg. She was observed for 15 months off treatment without problems or clinical recurrence.

Comments
Any fluid or pus collection in an ethnic-minority patient should be regarded as possibly tuberculous, even though the site appears unusual. The usual features of infection, namely redness, marked swelling and local heat, are not present – the so-called 'cold abscess'. Drug resistance may well be higher in such ethnic-minority groups, and a four-drug initial phase, including ethambutol, should be used to cover this eventuality. When isoniazid resistance is confirmed, the balance of opinion is that it should be removed from the regimen, and a continuation phase of rifampicin/ethambutol should be used for at least a further 7 months. However, in Third World settings, where drug sensitivity testing is seldom available, there is some evidence of a low relapse rate with standard short-course chemotherapy, provided that the initial phase is adequate.

Reference
Joint Tuberculosis Committee of the British Thoracic Society. 1998: Chemotherapy and management of tuberculosis in the United Kingdom: recommendations 1998. *Thorax* **53**, 536–48.

Cross reference
Chapter 4, Drug resistance

Case 61   A swelling in the breast

Presenting complaint
A 25-year-old Indian woman was seen with a swelling in the axillary tail of the right breast.

History of presenting complaint
The patient had been in the UK for 6 years and had made no return visits to India. She had been aware of some intermittent discomfort in the area of the axillary tail of the right breast for 2 years, but had only been aware of a palpable swelling for 2 months. She had not lost weight, but had felt 'hot' and had a dry cough intermittently.

Past medical history
There was no past medical history of note.

Examination
There was a fluctuant swelling in the tail of the right breast. No other abnormalities were found.

Tests
Haemoglobin was 10.0 g/dL, MCV was 64 fL and ESR was 57 mm/h. Haemoglobin electrophoresis showed beta-thalassaemia minor. The tuberculin test was strongly positive. Aspiration of the lesion yielded 50 mL of turbid fluid. Cytology and standard culture were negative, and AFB culture was requested. Chest X-ray was suggestive of right paratracheal lymphadenopathy (Fig. 61.1).

Progress
The patient was referred to the chest service by her surgeon with a clinical diagnosis of a tuberculous breast abscess. Treatment was commenced with Rifater and ethambutol (15 mg/kg). Weekly aspirations were needed in addition for a few weeks, but the volume aspirated declined over 4 weeks from 60 mL to 5 mL, and only one further aspiration was needed after a further 2 weeks. Itching from the medication was a problem, but there was no rash, and liver function was normal. The itching was controlled by concomitant administration of terfenadine 60 mg bd. By 2 months there was no palpable abnormality in the breast, the chest X-ray had returned to normal, and fully sensitive M. tuberculosis had been grown from the initial aspirate. Pyrazinamide and ethambutol were stopped and treatment was completed with 4 months of rifampicin/isoniazid.

Comment
Here again the features of a cold abscess, albeit in an unusual position, alerted the surgeon to the likelihood of tuberculosis. Such cold abscesses, as with lymph-node abscesses, may require regular aspiration in the initial few weeks, but the

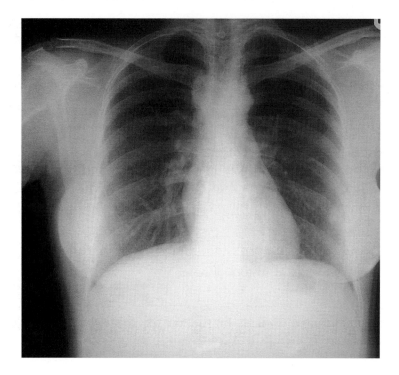

Fig. 61.1

volume and purulence of the aspirate usually decline rapidly. This abscess had no discharge through the skin, and no nipple discharge. Other forms of tuberculous breast disease have to be considered in ethnic-minority groups. Tuberculosis of the breast can also present as a mass simulating carcinoma, or as an abscess discharging through the nipple. One of the authors has seen a case in which a 2-month-old child presented with miliary tuberculosis, the mother having a normal chest X-ray but a breast abscess, with M. *tuberculosis* grown from the milk expressed from that side. The pruritis, which was thought to be due to pyrazinamide, was controlled by antihistamines, so allowing a 6-month regimen to be used. Removal of the pyrazinamide would have meant that a 9-month regimen of rifampicin/isoniazid supplemented by 2 months of initial ethambutol would be required.

Cross reference
Chapter 2, Management of adverse drug reactions

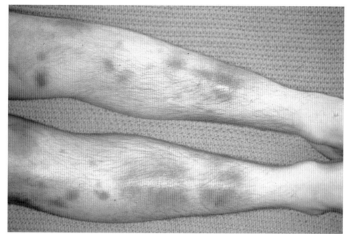
Plate 7.1

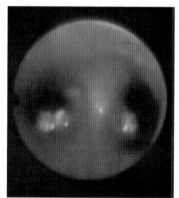
Plate 14.1

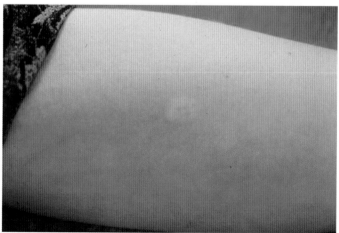
Plate 15.1

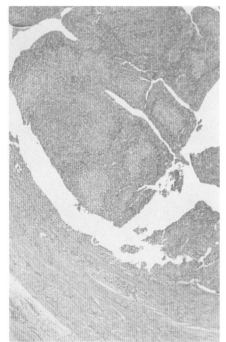

Plate 27.1

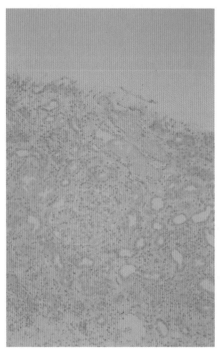

Plate 28.1

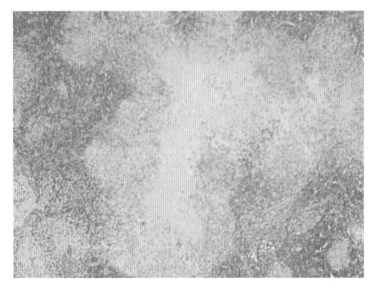

Plate 50.1 Haematoxylin and eosin (HE) stain of mediastinal gland biopsy showing poorly formed granulomata.

Plate 50.2 The same biopsy with Ziehl-Nielsen (ZN) staining showing numerous bacilli.

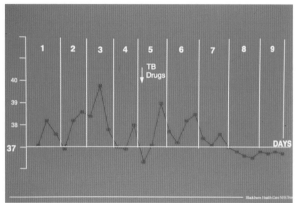

Plate 68.1

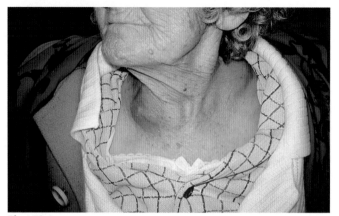

Plate 70.1

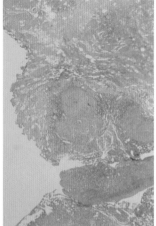

Plate 76.1

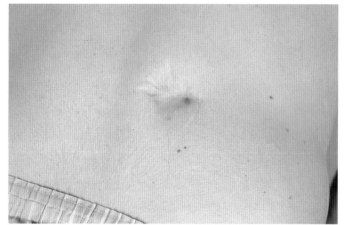

Plate 77.1

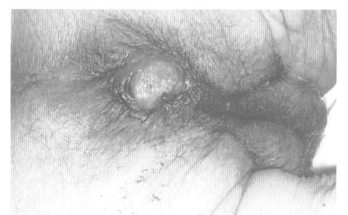

Plate 82.1

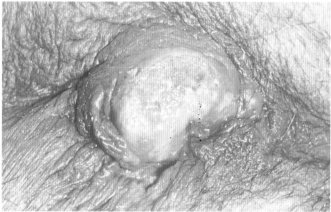

Plate 82.2

Plate 85.1

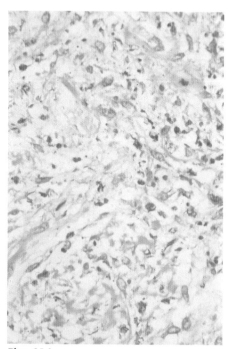

Plate 85.2

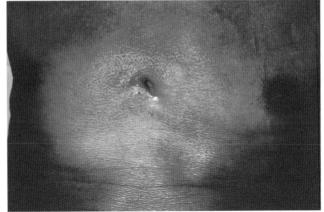

Plate 86.1

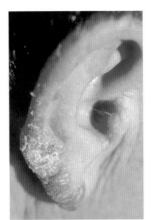

Plate 87.1

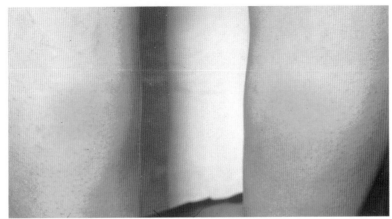

Plate 88.1

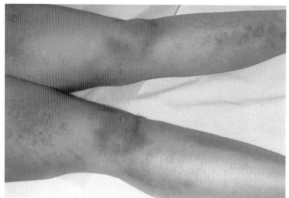

Plate 89.1

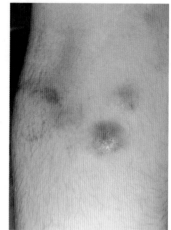

Plate 113.1

Plate 116.1 Reproduced courtesy of Dr. W. Taylor, Aintree University Hospital.

SECTION 6F CENTRAL NERVOUS SYSTEM DISEASE

Case 62   The feverish Pakistani

Presenting complaint
A 28-year-old Pakistani man presented with fever and malaise.

History of presenting complaint
The patient had been living in the UK for 3 years and had been feeling unwell with mild myalgia and fever for 2 months. He had had no headache, photophobia or respiratory symptoms. There was no past medical history of note.

Examination
The patient was febrile at 38.5°C, there were no focal signs in the chest, and there was no lymphadenopathy, hepatosplenomegaly, neck stiffness or photophobia.

Tests
Chest X-ray and abdominal ultrasound were normal. Haemoglobin was 11.4 g/dL with normal indices and normal WCC and platelets. Apart from sodium, which was low at 123 mmol/L, electrolytes were normal. A lumbar puncture was performed which showed a protein concentration of 1.94 g/L, a glucose level of 1.5 mmol/L and a WBC of 83 cells/mL, of which 90 per cent were mononuclear. CSF was sent for polymerase chain reaction (PCR) analysis for tuberculosis and was reported to be negative. Gram and ZN stains were negative.

Progress
In-patient retreatment was started with Rifater and ethambutol (15 mg/kg) (the patient's weight was 54.4 kg). Swinging fever persisted for 2 weeks, when repeat lumbar puncture showed a protein concentration of 1.83 g/L, a glucose level of 2.9 mmol/L and a WBC of 70 cells/mL. Liver function was normal and a CT brain scan showed no significant ventriculopathy. Prednisolone (50 mg/day) was added and treatment was continued. Although weight gain occurred, the fever persisted. The CSF was culture positive at 4 weeks in Kirschner medium. The fever resolved in the fifth week of treatment. All four antituberculosis drugs were continued until sensitivity results were available. These showed the organism to be highly resistant to isoniazid. By this stage, 2 months of treatment had been given. Pyrazinamide and isoniazid were stopped. Rifampicin (600 mg) and ethambutol (1000 mg) (patient's weight now 65 kg) were given under supervision. Six months into treatment a small fluctuant gland developed in the left supraclavicular fossa. A total of 5 mL of pus was aspirated but the aspirate was negative on culture. The gland settled over a few months with unaltered treatment. Treatment was stopped after 12 months.

Comment

The early stages of tuberculous meningitis can be non-specific, and not all cases have headache, photophobia or even fever. A high index of suspicion and early diagnosis are important as prognosis depends on the stage of disease. Cases without focal neurological signs or clouding of consciousness (Stage I) have a better prognosis than those with either focal neurological signs or clouding of consciousness (Stage II), which in turn have a much better prognosis than those in coma (Stage III). A completely normal lumbar puncture effectively excludes tuberculous meningitis. Although PCR for mycobacteria can be performed on CSF, there is a false-negative rate due to inhibitors in the CSF, and where the CSF pattern is consistent with tuberculous meningitis, even if no AFB are seen on microscopy, antituberculosis drugs should be given even if the PCR is negative. In this case the fever took a long time to settle, even with the administration of steroids for several weeks in addition. This was the first sign that the patient's progress was not straightforward, and since drug reaction and intracerebral complications had been excluded as causes of fever, it raised the possibility of drug resistance, which was later confirmed. Because of the meningitis and drug resistance, treatment was closely supervised. Progress was further complicated by the development of a sterile fluctuant node at 6 months, which resolved without alteration of the treatment regimen. The development of new nodes, or enlargement of pre-existing nodes, with or without fluctuation, occurs in up to 20 per cent of cases of peripheral lymphadenopathy, but less commonly with other forms of extrapulmonary disease. Such events do not in themselves suggest inadequate treatment, and if they are culture negative are thought to represent immunological events related to tuberculin positivity.

Reference

Humphries, M.J., Teoh, R., Law, J. and Gabriel, M. 1990: Factors of prognostic significance in Chinese children with tuberculous meningitis. *Tubercle* **71**, 161–8.

Cross references

Chapter 4, Drug resistance; Chapter 6, Section 6J, Lymph-node disease

Case 63   The confused housewife

Presenting complaint
A 43-year-old Pakistani housewife presented with a history of headaches for 2 months and confusion for 1 week.

History of presenting complaint
The patient had lived in the UK for 9 years, and had made one return visit to Pakistan 30 months earlier. She had experienced headaches for 2 months, accompanied by weight loss of 12 kg. For the previous week she had been confused and she had also complained of intermittent double vision. There was no past medical history of relevance.

Examination
The patient was afebrile, but was disorientated with regard to time and place. There were no long tract signs or papilloedema, but there was an intermittent internuclear ophthalmoplegia.

Tests
Chest X-ray was normal, and sodium was 128 mmol/L. CT brain scan was normal. A lumbar puncture showed a CSF glucose concentration of 1.2 mmol/L (blood 7.1 mmol/L), protein 4.9 g/L and WCC of 15×10^6/mL, all mononuclear. Gram and ZN stains were negative.

Progress
The patient was started on Rifater and prothionamide (visual acuity could not be assessed, and prothionamide penetrates CSF better than either streptomycin or ethambutol), and dexamethasone 4 mg tds. After 2 weeks her balance deteriorated, with left-sided minor cerebellar signs and a partial right third nerve palsy. Repeat CT scan showed minimal ventricular dilatation and a developing left thalamic tuberculoma. Treatment was continued with some improvement, but the diplopia persisted. A 8 weeks M. *tuberculosis* was cultured from the initial CSF, and when full sensitivity was confirmed 3 weeks later, pyrazinamide and prothionamide were stopped. Treatment with rifampicin/isoniazid was continued, and dexamethasone was slowly withdrawn. A CT scan at 5 months showed no mass but slightly reduced attenuation in the right posterior parietal/ occipital areas. After 9 months the patient became more confused and had brisk left-sided reflexes. A CT scan (Fig. 63.1) showed a large right temporoparietal lesion with oedema. The appearances were more suggestive of tumour than of tuberculoma, and a neurosurgical biopsy was performed which showed tuberculoma. Dexamethasone was reintroduced and treatment was continued with rifampicin and isoniazid. The lesion gradually improved on CT. Drug treatment was stopped after 17 months. The patient has been left with altered personality, a mild left-sided weakness and diplopia, the latter corrected by refraction.

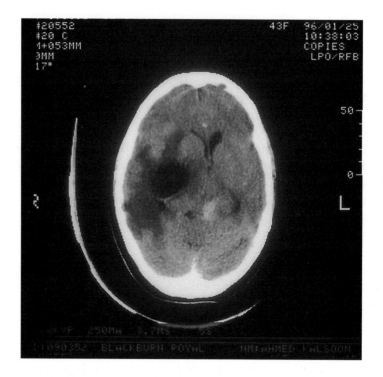

Fig. 63.1

Comment

In this case tuberculous meningitis was suspected even though there was no fever. This was at Stage II with focal neurological signs and altered consciousness, so corticosteroids were also given. A CT scan of the brain was initially normal, but the development of tuberculomas during treatment and the paradoxical enlargement of existing tuberculomas during treatment are both well documented. Neurosurgical intervention is seldom required for tuberculomas but is occasionally required for pressure effects, or to make a diagnosis when the appearance on CT scan is not classic and a tumour is in the differential diagnosis. In such circumstances treatment may need to be prolonged beyond 12 months. Outcome is related to stage at diagnosis, with Stage I having a high cure rate with low morbidity and mortality. Stage II disease has a higher mortality and residual morbidity in 20 per cent of cases. Stage III disease has a mortality approaching 80 per cent, and all survivors have some degree of handicap.

Reference

Teoh, I.R., Humphries, M.J. and O'Mahoney, G. 1987: Symptomatic intracranial tuberculoma developing during treatment of tuberculosis – a report of 10 cases and a review of the literature. *Quarterly Journal of Medicine* **241**, 449–60.

Case 64   Malaise and headaches

Presenting complaint
A 29-year-old Indian man presented with a history of malaise for 2 months and headache for 1 week.

History of presenting complaint
The patient had been living in the UK for 18 months, had made no return visits to India, and had experienced fever, mainly at night, for 2 months. In the preceding week he had developed a headache without photophobia or vomiting. There was no past medical history of note.

Examination
The patient was febril up to 39°C, fundal examination was normal and there was no neck stiffness.

He had a soft apical systolic murmur. There were no signs in the lungs, and no lymphadenopathy or hepatosplenomegaly.

Tests
An initial chest X-ray that was a little over-penetrated appeared normal (Fig. 64.1). Echocardiogram showed minor mitral valve prolapse and no vegetations.

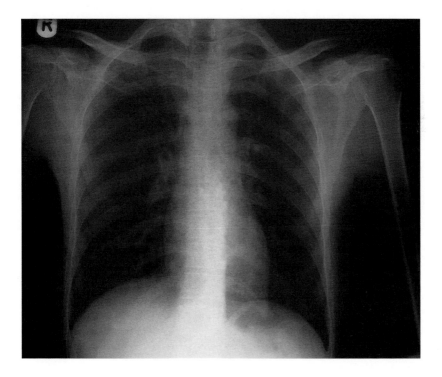

Fig. 64.1

ESR was 16 mm/h and globulin was 37 g/L. Lumbar puncture showed a protein concentration of 1.93 g/L, a glucose concentration of 0.6 mmol/L and a WBC of 131 cells/mL with 60 per cent monocytosis. Gram and ZN stains were negative.

Progress

A presumptive diagnosis of tuberculous meningitis was made and treatment with Rifater and ethambutol (15 mg/kg) was commenced (patient's weight was 42.9 kg). Chest X-ray was repeated and, with a softer film (Fig. 64.2; high detail from right mid zone), early miliary disease was apparent. A CT brain scan showed no evidence of tuberculomas or hydrocephalus. By 2 months the chest X-ray had returned to normal and the patient had gained 7 kg. The drug dosage was adjusted upwards for weight gain. A positive culture for M. *tuberculosis* was obtained at 8 weeks.

The four drugs were continued until full sensitivity of the organism was confirmed. Pyrazinamide and ethambutol were then stopped, and rifampicin/ isoniazid were continued for a total of 12 months.

Comment

Tuberculous meningitis complicates up to 30 per cent of cases of miliary tuberculosis. If there is a miliary pattern on chest X-ray, a lumbar puncture has

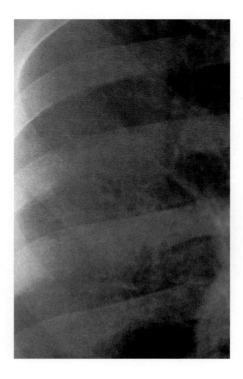

Fig. 64.2

a significant yield even in the absence of symptoms. Miliary disease may be missed if the chest X-ray is over-penetrated, and is seen better on a 'soft' film. Alternatively, the initial chest X-ray may be normal and the miliary pattern may only be seen on a later film. Patients often gain substantial amounts of weight during treatment, and dosages of antituberculosis drugs may need to be increased during treatment if this occurs.

Reference
Ormerod, L.P. and Horsfield, N. 1995: Miliary tuberculosis in a high prevalence area of the United Kingdom: Blackburn 1978–93. *Respiratory Medicine* **89**, 555–7.

Case 65   Weight loss in an Asian woman

Presenting complaint
A 21-year-old Asian woman was seen with weight loss, fever and cough.

History of presenting complaint
The patient had given birth 4 months earlier when her weight was 44 kg postpartum. Since the birth she had lost over 10 kg, and she had had night sweats and fevers.

Past medical history
The patient had arrived from India 2 years earlier and had no other medical history of note.

Examination
The patient was very thin and wasted (weight 30.5 kg), with a fever of 38.6°C, and occasional crackles only in the chest.

Tests
Chest X-ray showed infiltration in both mid and upper zones with early cavitation (Fig. 65.1). She was too weak to be able to cough up secretions, so a

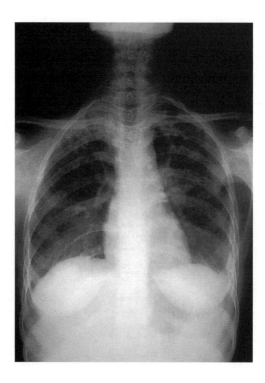

Fig. 65.1

fibre-optic bronchoscopy was performed with bilateral upper zone washings for AFB microscopy and culture. Treatment was started immediately with prednisolone (30 mg/day), Rifater (3 tablets) and ethambutol (500 mg). Secretions from both lungs were heavily smear positive for AFB. The patient improved over 4 weeks in hospital, gaining 7 kg in weight and tolerating treatment. She was allowed home, but was readmitted the following day after a single convulsion. A CT brain scan (Fig. 65.2) showed a 1-cm parietal tuberculoma. Carbamezepine (100 mg bd) was added to her treatment.

M. *tuberculosis* that was fully sensitive to first-line drugs was grown from the patient's bronchoscopy washings. Pyrazinamide and ethambutol were stopped after 8 weeks. A repeat brain scan after 6 months showed that the parietal lesion was still present. It was planned to perform a further CT scan after 12 months of treatment with a view to stopping treatment at that time, but the patient became pregnant after 9 months of treatment, so this was postponed until she was postpartum again (17 months). The repeat CT then showed resolution, and rifampicin/isoniazid were stopped.

Comment

There were no signs or symptoms of CNS involvement in this young woman, who did, however, have very extensive pulmonary disease. At presentation her 4-month-old baby was put on isoniazid syrup (5 mg/kg) until serial tuberculin tests were shown to be negative, on the assumption that the mother would have

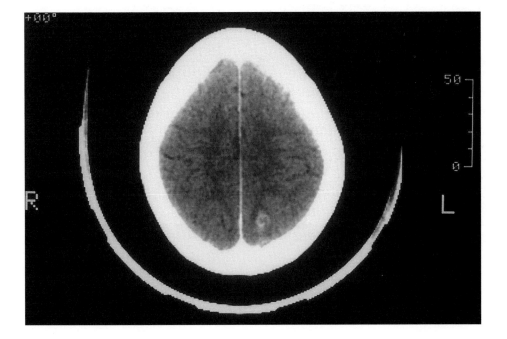

Fig. 65.2

been smear positive on sputum before she became too weak to expectorate. The finding of CNS disease altered treatment with regard to duration. Treatment was prolonged beyond 6 months because of the CNS involvement, and was planned to stop at 12 months. The treatment was prolonged through the patient's second pregnancy, as we did not want to give excessive radiation (CT of the brain) during pregnancy. The child, who had been conceived while the patient was on rifampicin/isoniazid, was normal. The treatment of tuberculosis in pregnancy is the same as standard treatment, apart from two small differences. None of the first-line drugs is teratogenic, but streptomycin should be avoided as it is ototoxic to the fetus. If second-line or reserve drugs have to be used, ethionamide and prothionamide should be avoided, as they are potentially teratogenic.

Reference
Lees, A.J., Macleod, A.F. and Marshall, J. 1980: Cerebral tuberculomas developing during treatment of tuberculous meningitis. *Lancet* **i**, 1208–11.

Case 66   All boxed in

Presenting complaint
A 25-year-old woman was admitted to hospital in Pakistan with a history of dry cough, night sweats, malaise and loss of 7 kg in weight over a period of 2 months.

History of presenting complaint
She worked in a factory making cardboard boxes, and had recently noticed difficulty in using her right hand.

Examination
On examination she was found to have a left-sided pleural effusion. No neurological abnormalities were noted at this time.

Tests
The Mantoux test was strongly positive (22 mm in duration to 10 TU) and the chest radiograph revealed bilateral pulmonary infiltration and left-sided pleural effusion.

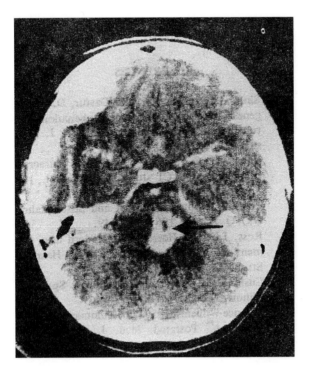

Fig. 66.1

Progress

The patient was started on standard quadruple therapy of rifampicin (10 mg/kg), isoniazid (300 mg/day), ethambutol (15 mg/kg) and pyrazinamide (30 mg/kg). There was a good clinical response with improvement in cough and appetite, but the patient developed chorioathetoid movements in her right hand 3 weeks after the chemotherapy was started. A CT scan showed an ill-defined low-density mass extending from the pons almost to the quadrigeminal plate on the left distortion of the fourth ventricle. After contrast there was irregular ring enhancement of this lesion (Fig. 66.1). A further enhancing area was identified in the left parietal region near the vertex and central sulcus (Fig. 66.2). A diagnosis of intracranial tuberculomas was made. The dose of chemotherapy was increased to rifampicin 20 mg/kg and ethambutol 25 mg/kg body weight.

The patient's neurological symptoms continued to progress, and she developed twitching of her right leg, pyramidal signs on the right side and an upper motor neurone facial nerve palsy which was assumed to be due to paradoxical expansion of the tuberculomas. The treatment was continued and 2 months after increasing the dose of chemotherapy an improvement in neurological signs was observed. After 6 months the patient complained only of occasional twitching of her arm. A repeat CT scan at this stage showed a dramatic reduction in the size of the lesions (Figs 66.3 and 66.4).

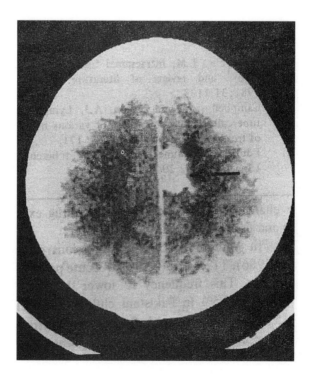

Fig. 66.2

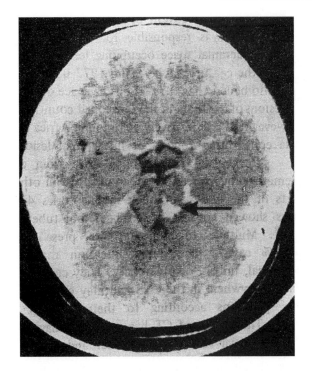

Fig. 66.3

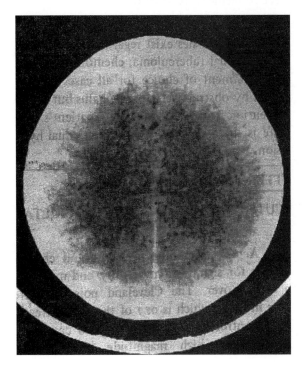

Fig. 66.4

Comment

In this patient two unsuspected tuberculomas were confirmed on CT scan, after which neurological signs had appeared following the start of chemotherapy for pulmonary tuberculosis. The signs continued to deteriorate for 2 months despite increasing the doses as is usually recommended for tuberculosis of the brain.

Intracranial tuberculoma is common in the Indian subcontinent. The incidence of intracranial tuberculoma has declined since the advent of effective treatment. At the turn of the century tuberculosis was responsible for about 30 to 40 per cent of all intracranial-space-occupying lesions, whereas in 1972 it was estimated to be linked with less than 0.5 per cent of all the space-occupying lesions of the brain in the developed countries. However, it is still relatively common in Africa and Asia, representing 16.20 per cent of intracranial lesions.

Intracranial tuberculomas arise from the haematogenous spread of tuberculosis from other parts of the body, although in one study 42 per cent of cases showed no signs of extracerebral tuberculosis. Multiple tuberculomas are present in 15.34 per cent of cases. The initial infection may be meningeal, miliary or pulmonary. These tuberculomas can occur almost anywhere in the CNS, and may cause pressure problems, depending on their location.

The advent of CT has made the diagnosis of intracranial tuberculomas easier and provides much clearer details of the anatomical site. It is also helpful for evaluating the effect of medical treatment.

There is controversy regarding the treatment of intracranial tuberculoma. Chemotherapy alone may be sufficient, but when complicated by obstructive hydrocephalus, surgical intervention is indicated, especially when the patient's vision is threatened by severe intracranial hypertension.

SECTION 6G MILIARY DISEASE

Case 67 White cryptic disease

Presenting complaint
A 37-year-old white man presented with a 3-week history of fever and malaise.

History of presenting complaint
The patient had been well until the previous 3 weeks, and had not travelled overseas. He had lost 7 kg in weight and had experienced some sweats. He had lost his appetite but had no respiratory or CNS symptoms. There was no past medical history of note.

Examination
The patient's weight was 76 kg. There were no physical signs, and he was febrile at 38.5°C.

Tests
Chest X-ray was normal. Haemoglobin was 12.3 g/dL, ESR was 109 mm/h, C-reactive protein (CRP) was 33.5 U/L (normal range < 7 U/L) and WBC was 4.3 × 10^6/mL. Ultrasound of the abdomen and autoantibodies were normal. Blood cultures were taken and the patient was given Ceftiaxone intravenously for 7 days. He continued to experience fever up to 38.5°C. Serial virology was negative, and echocardiogram and immunoglobulins were normal. The tuberculin test was negative. The fever appeared to settle somewhat after 2 weeks, and ESR was 59 mm/h.

Progress
The patient was allowed home with temperature monitoring. At review at 4 and 8 weeks he was still experiencing intermittent pyrexia to 38°C, and had lost a further 4 kg. Physical examination was again normal. He was readmitted and reinvestigated as a case of pyrexia of unknown origin. ESR was 58–75 mm/h, haemoglobin was 10.9 g/dL normochromic, and liver function was again normal. A CT scan of the abdomen and chest X-ray were both normal. Brucella and Widal were normal, and bone marrow showed secondary anaemia only. Autoantibodies and a vasculitis screen were negative. The tuberculin test was negative, and the patient's temperature continued up to 38.5°C

After negative investigations over 2 weeks, and with a total period of 15 weeks of fever, the patient was given a trial of antituberculosis treatment with Rifater 6 tablets. His fever settled in 7 days, and this was maintained on home recordings over the next 2 months. He gained 3 kg in 2 weeks and 7 kg in 2 months. The ESR had fallen to 2 mm/h by 2 months. Repeat tuberculin testing was now strongly positive. Treatment with Rifinah 300 was given for a further 4 months. The patient gained 13.5 kg overall, and haemoglobin was 14.9 g/dL normochromic and ESR was 7 mm/h at the end of treatment. He remained well over 12 months of follow-up with no recurrence of symptoms.

Comment

Because he was a white, previously healthy young man with no HIV risk factors, an underlying lymphoma or collagen disease was initially considered likely. The tuberculin test was twice negative and there was never any bacteriological or histological evidence of tuberculosis. After many weeks of negative investigations, but continuing gradual weight loss, fever and raised ESR, a trial of antituberculosis treatment was given, with de-fervescence in 7 days, together with a striking weight gain and fall in ESR over 2 months. If the patient had been of ethnic-minority extraction, a trial of antituberculosis treatment would have been given much earlier because of the much higher probability of tuberculosis, and hence the higher index of suspicion. The tuberculin test can be negative in cases of disseminated miliary (cryptic) tuberculosis, and may only become positive after 6 to 8 weeks of treatment. Ideally, rifampicin should not be included in a trial of antituberculosis treatment, as occult Gram-negative infection could respond, whereas isoniazid, pyrazinamide and ethambutol are purely antimycobacterial drugs. In practical terms, however, the benefits of using combination tablets with the three main bactericidal antituberculosis drugs all included outweigh this theoretical consideration. In high-prevalence, low-income countries a trial of treatment after exclusion of pneumonia, malaria and enteric fever may be all that is available.

Case 68 An Asian case of pyrexia of unknown origin

Presenting complaint
A 23-year-old Indian housewife was referred with night sweats and weight loss.

History of presenting complaint
The patient had been in the UK for 7 months, and her mother had had tuberculosis in the past in India. She complained of weight loss of 7 kg and some night sweats and fever for 2 weeks. She had had ampicillin without effect, apart from causing a rash.

Examination
Apart from a weight of 35.6 kg and a fever of 38.5°C there were no abnormalities on examination.

Tests
Haemoglobin was 10.7 g/dL, MCV was 74.9 fL and ESR was 76 mm/h. Liver function was normal but globulin was raised at 42 g/L. Blood cultures and blood for malaria parasites were negative. A chest X-ray and barium meal and follow-through were normal. The sputum samples were negative on microscopy. Three EMU samples were sent. The tuberculin test was moderately positive (Heaf grade 3).

Progress
Because of continuing swinging fever (Plate 68.1) and negative investigations, after appropriate bacteriology samples had been sent a trial of antituberculosis treatment with rifampicin, isoniazid and pyrazinamide (as Rifater) was given. The fever responded within 3 days. The patient gained weight rapidly and within 2 weeks had reached 40 kg, requiring the dosage of antituberculosis medication to be increased. After 2 months of treatment the haemoglobin was 12.6 g/dL normochromic and the ESR was 25 mm/h. Sputum and urine cultures were negative for M. tuberculosis. Pyrazinamide was stopped, and rifampicin/isoniazid were given for a further 4 months. The patient's final weight was 46 kg.

Comment
Because of her ethnic origin, age and previous history of tuberculosis contact, an early trial of antituberculosis drugs was performed. The fever responded rapidly in this case, but may take between 7 and 14 days to settle in other cases. Weight gain may require adjustment of drug dosages during treatment. In such cases a liver biopsy may show granulomata and allow a positive culture. In Third World countries only a trial of drugs with monitoring of fever and body weight may be possible. Such cases of disseminated tuberculosis with normal examination and

chest X-ray are sometimes described as 'cryptic miliary' as they have a hidden source, to differentiate them from cases with a diffusely abnormal X-ray – the 'classical miliary' cases.

Reference
Proudfoot, A.T. 1971: Cryptic disseminated tuberculosis. *British Journal of Hospital Medicine* **5**, 773–80.

Case 69   A wasted febrile old man

Presenting complaint
An 82-year-old Pakistani man with weight loss, malaise and sweats was seen by a geriatrician.

History of presenting complaint
The patient had first come to the UK 3 years earlier, but had had a recent 4-month stay in Pakistan. He had lost in excess of 5 kg, had a poor appetite and had had sweats and fevers for 1 month. Six months earlier while in Pakistan he had fallen on to his sternum, and he had subsequently developed a swelling near the xipihisterum which he attributed to this fall.

Past medical history
The patient had reduced visual acuity due to bilateral cataracts.

Examination
The patient was thin at 47 kg, febrile at 38.2°C and had a fluctuant swelling with some erythema just lateral to the xiphisternum on the right.

Tests
ESR was 54 mm/h and globulin was 44 g/L. Chest X-ray showed right apical pleural scarring and miliary shadowing (Fig. 69.1). Liver function and ultrasound of the abdomen were normal. The fluctuant lesion was aspirated and 3 mL of pus were sent for AFB culture.

Progress
Based on the chest X-ray and what was clinically considered to be a subcutaneous tuberculosis abscess, treatment was commenced with rifampicin, isoniazid and pyrazinamide. Ethambutol was not given because of the patient's reduced visual acuity. Some nausea was experienced with the tablets, but liver function was normal. The nausea was controlled by metoclopramide as needed. A sinus developed at the site of aspiration, which was treated with twice-weekly dressings. The fever settled in 1 week. After 2 months the miliary shadowing had substantially cleared on X-ray, and the sinus healed by granulation from the base. The pus was positive for M. tuberculosis which was fully sensitive. At 2 months the patient's weight was 50.7 kg. Pyrazinamide was stopped and rifampicin/isoniazid were given for a further 4 months. The patient's final weight was 58.5 kg.

Comment
The symptoms other than the soft-tissue abscess were non-specific, and no respiratory symptoms were observed. The soft-tissue abscess allowed a rapid diagnosis and enabled bacteriology results to be obtained. If there had been no

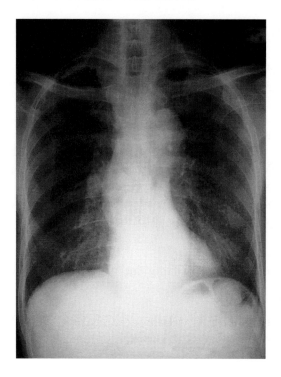

Fig. 69.1

soft-tissue abscess, a lumbar puncture might have given bacteriology results, as up to 30 per cent of cases with 'classical' miliary shadowing have associated meningitis even in the absence of symptoms. Ideally, a fourth drug would have been used because of the higher rate of drug resistance in such cases, but ethambutol was contraindicated due to the patient's poor visual acuity, and streptomycin was also contraindicated because of the greatly increased likelihood of oto- or nephrotoxicity at this age.

Reference
Ormerod, L.P. and Horsfield, N. 1995: Miliary tuberculosis in a high prevalence area of the United Kingdom: Blackburn 1978–93. *Respiratory Medicine* **89**, 555–7.

Case 70   A wasted old woman

Presenting complaint
An 88-year-old white woman was brought to the clinic by her sister from another area. She complained of weight loss and bilateral neck swellings.

History of presenting complaint
The patient had been losing weight for several months, and weighed 41.3 kg. Neck swellings had been present bilaterally for 6 weeks and were increasing in size. Her sister suspected malignancy.

Past medical history
No major past illnesses or operations were elicited.

Examination
The patient was thin. There were bilateral swellings in both supraclavicular fossae, and these were more marked on the right with fluctuation (Plate 70.1).

Tests
The surgeon suspected cold abscesses and aspirated the right swelling, obtaining pus. Chest X-ray (Fig. 70.1) showed miliary tuberculosis and bilateral soft-tissue swellings in the neck. ESR was 20 mm/h. The patient was seen the same day by the chest service, and 20 mL of pus were aspirated from the left neck swelling and a further 70 mL of pus from the right neck swelling. These aspirates, together with EMUs and sputum samples were sent for tuberculosis culture.

Progress
The patient was started on Rifater and pyridoxine, and the neck required bilateral aspirations weekly for 5 weeks. A sinus developed on the left side which required packing until it healed by granulation over a period of 3 months. Initial liver function was normal, but after 5 weeks the patient developed malaise and anorexia but no vomiting. Bilirubin was 30 g/L and ALT was 380 IU/L. Rifampicin, isoniazid and pyrazinamide were stopped, but because the patient was still ill and had disseminated disease, treatment with ethambutol (15 mg/kg) and ofloxacin (400 mg bd) was given until the ALT activity returned to normal. Isoniazid was reintroduced at 50 mg/day for 3 days, and then at 300 mg daily, followed by rifampicin at 150 mg/day for 3 days and then 450 mg daily, with liver function monitoring, which remained normal. Ofloxacin was then stopped and treatment continued with rifampicin/isoniazid and ethambutol for 2 months, followed by rifampicin/isoniazid for a further 6 months. Cultures of fully sensitive M. *tuberculosis* were obtained from the neck pus, sputum and EMU samples after 4 weeks.

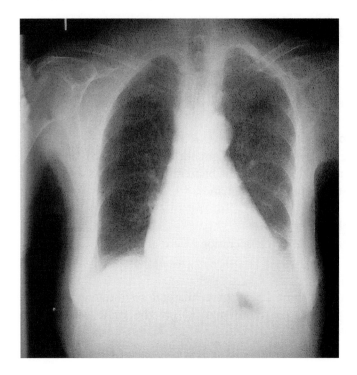

Fig. 70.1

Comment

Miliary disease presented here as weight loss without fever and neck masses (which were cold abscesses) simulating malignancy. There were no respiratory or urinary symptoms, but positive cultures were obtained from these sites. The lymph-node abscesses required regular initial aspirations and were complicated by the development of a sinus. This resolved with packing (to allow healing by granulation from the base) and standard drug treatment. The incidence of drug-induced hepatitis increases with age, and is higher in women. Because the patient had disseminated disease, she was treated with two non-hepatotoxic drugs (ethambutol and ofloxacin) until isoniazid and rifampicin had been successfully reintroduced. In the white population the incidence of miliary disease is highest at the extremes of age.

Reference

British Thoracic Society Research Committee. 1992: Six-months versus nine-months chemotherapy for tuberculosis of lymph nodes: preliminary results. *Respiratory Medicine* **83**, 15–19.

Case 71   The pneumoconiosis that never was

Presenting complaint
A 60-year-old former miner was admitted with general deterioration and vague chest pain.

History of presenting complaint
The patient lived alone and drank to excess (> 50 units of alcohol/week). He had been losing weight and had experienced malaise for 2 months. He also had vague non-localized chest pain and a dry cough.

Past medical history
The patient gave a history of having been diagnosed with coal-miner's pneumoconiosis.

Examination
The patient had a low-grade fever (37.8°C), a sinus tachycardia at 110 beats/min, and a palpable liver (two fingers). There were no crackles or focal signs in the chest.

Tests
Haemoglobin was 15.1 g/dL with an MCV of 103 fL. The platelet count was 98 $\times 10^6$/mL and WCC was 3.7 $\times 10^6$/mL. Sodium was 128 mmol/L, albumen was 26 g/dL and gamma glutamyl transferase (GT) was 436 IU/L. Bone marrow showed normal maturation of all entities and no megaloblastic change. A chest X-ray (Fig. 71.1) showed diffuse nodular shadowing thought to be consistent with the patient's history of pneumoconiosis.

Progress
The patient continued to run a low-grade fever between 37 and 38°C, and was investigated as a case of pyrexia of unknown origin over 3 weeks. An abdominal ultrasound scan showed fatty infiltration of the liver only. Autoantibodies and a collagen screen were negative. The chest service was contacted for advice. The patient had been seen 3 years earlier because he believed he had a pneumo-coniosis, but the chest X-ray had been entirely normal (Fig. 71.2). Because of the fever, X-ray changes and low white cell count, disseminated tuberculosis was suspected. Sputum was sent for microscopy and was 2+ positive for AFBs. Treatment with Rifater and prednisolone (50 mg/day) was started with weekly liver-function monitoring in view of the patient's alcoholism. A further complication was an ultrasound-proven ileofemoral thrombosis treated with warfarin. The patient showed a slow improvement with the above treatment, with pyridoxine (vitamin B_6) 10 mg/day and thiamine (vitamin B_1) 100 mg/day. After 2 months of treatment his chest X-ray was virtually normal. Sputum grew M. *tuberculosis* that was fully sensitive to first-line drugs. Warfarin and

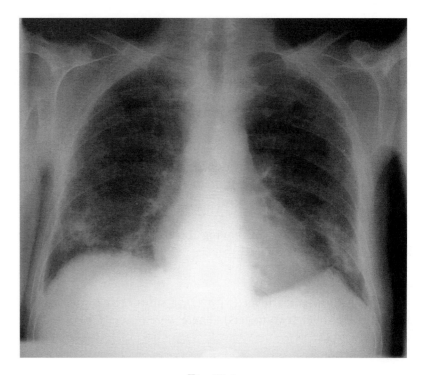

Fig. 71.1

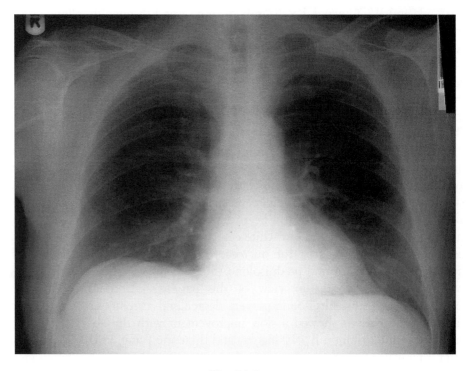

Fig. 71.2

pyrazinamide were stopped on discharge after 2 months. Steroids were withdrawn over the first 3 months. Treatment with rifampicin/isoniazid and pyridoxine was given for a further 4 months on a daily basis supervised by a family member. The patient gained 19 kg over the 6-month treatment period.

Comment

In this case the initial medical team was led astray by the incorrect history of pneumoconiosis. With an abnormal X-ray it is always worth examining previous films where these exist. This allowed the correct diagnosis to be suspected, and it was immediately confirmed by sputum examination. Regular liver-function monitoring was carried out because of pre-existing alcohol-associated liver disease. Rifampicin can induce the metabolism of warfarin, with larger doses being needed and close coagulation control being required. The appearance of the chest X-ray was nearer that of a tuberculous bronchopneumonia than that of a true miliary pattern.

Cross references

Chapter 3, Patients with adverse risk factors; Chapter 11, Altered diagnosis

Case 72   Fever and right leg weakness in an Indian housewife

Presenting complaint
A 41-year-old, previously healthy housewife presented with a 2-month history of low-grade pyrexia (38.5°C in the axilla). The fever showed an evening rise and was accompanied by chills but no rigors.

History of presenting complaint
The patient denied any history of cough or headache, and had no past history of tuberculosis or contact with the disease. She had received empirical antimalarial medication and antibiotics, without any relief of her symptoms.

Examination and tests
Physical examination was normal. Haemoglobin was 13 g/dL, WCC was 7.1 × 10^6/mL with a normal differential, and ESR was 70 mm/h. Antinuclear antibody (ANA) blood and urine cultures were negative. Chest radiography and sonography of the abdomen and pelvis were normal. A high-resolution computerized tomography (HRCT) scan of the chest was performed, and this showed diffuse miliary shadowing (Fig. 72.1). As attempts at sputum induction were unsuccessful, a fibre-optic bronchoscopy was performed and a broncho-alveolar lavage (BAL) of the middle lobe was positive for AFB.

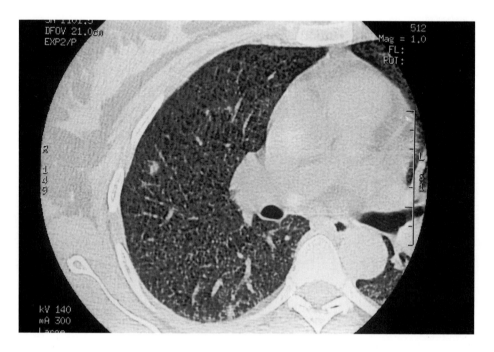

Fig. 72.1

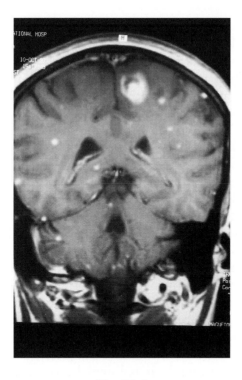

Fig. 72.2

Progress

The patient was commenced on standard four-drug antituberculosis therapy (isoniazid, rifampicin, pyrazinamide, ethambutol) (HRZE) and streptomycin together with 30 mg prednisolone. The latter was tapered off and stopped within 1 month. The patient's fever settled promptly, but 6 weeks after commencing her treatment she woke with acute weakness of the right leg severe enough to make her drag her leg whilst walking. This improved spontaneously over the next 7 days, and when seen at this stage she had a pure motor weakness of the right leg (4+ power) with brisk knee and ankle jerks. Magnetic resonance imaging (MRI) of the brain performed at this stage revealed multiple diffusely enhancing miliary lesions in both cerebral hemispheres, the cerebellum and brainstem, with some surrounding white-matter oedema. A larger ring-enhancing lesion 1.5 cm in diameter was seen in the left parasagittal cortex (Fig. 72.2).

Since the patient was improving spontaneously, no changes were made in her treatment and within 1 month her leg power had returned to normal. She went on to make a complete recovery.

Comment

Miliary tuberculosis is one of the commonest causes of pyrexia of unknown origin in India. It occurs when there is haematogenous dissemination of tuberculosis. Whilst fever is recognized as a cardinal symptom of miliary tuberculosis, what is less well known is that cough and dyspnoea may be absent in as many as 40 per cent of patients.

Physical examination may be normal, as it was in this patient. Choroid tubercles should always be diligently looked for, as they are specific for haematogenously disseminated tuberculosis but are found in no more than 5 per cent of all patients. They are probably frequently missed because dilatation with mydriatics is required. An autopsy study found choroid tubercles in 50 per cent of eyes examined.

The chest X-ray may be completely normal in about 15 per cent of patients with miliary tuberculosis, especially in the first few weeks of illness. HRCT is much more sensitive, but does not specifically distinguish miliary tuberculosis from other causes of miliary mottling. Bronchial washings have a diagnostic yield of about 80 per cent, and if transbronchial biopsies are performed at the time, the yield increases to 90 per cent.

Central nervous involvement in the form of meningitis or tuberculomas is recognized clinically in 15 to 30 per cent of patients with miliary tuberculosis. The real incidence may be much higher because involvement may be asymptomatic and therefore under-appreciated. In the patient described above the sudden neurological weakness indicated the presence of brain involvement. It is possible that withdrawing the initial steroid cover resulted in an increase in brain oedema and lesion size. Spontaneous expansion of intracranial tuberculomas while on treatment is also well documented.

Cross reference
Chapter 6, Section 6F, Central nervous system disease

Case 73　The nonagenarian

Presenting complaint
A 90–year-old woman was admitted with a 6-month history of anorexia and weight loss. She had had diarrhoea and confusion for 1 week.

History of presenting complaint
Six weeks previously she had been admitted for investigation of her symptoms. A diagnosis of non-insulin-dependent diabetes had been made, and she had been discharged on oral hypoglycaemic agents. In the week before her second admission she had become rapidly unwell.

Examination
At her second admission the patient was ill, confused and pyrexial (38.0°C), with a heart rate of 120 beats/min (atrial fibrillation), a blood pressure of 80/0 mmHg, and widespread crackles heard on chest auscultation.

Tests
The patient's chest X-ray at the first admission had shown clear lung fields and a hiatus hernia (Fig. 73.1). On the second admission there was widespread miliary shadowing (Fig. 73.2). The patient was hyponatraemic (122 mmol/L)

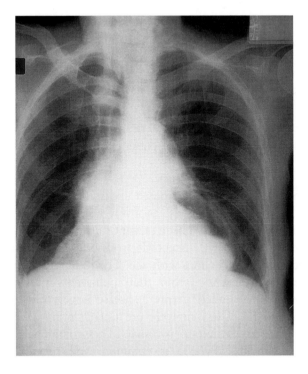

Fig. 73.1

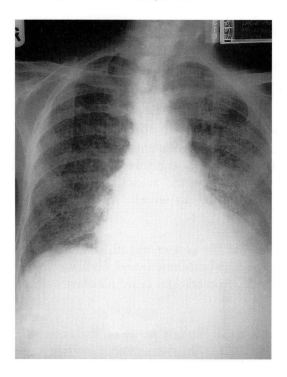

Fig. 73.2

with impaired renal function (urea 27.8 mmol/L, normal range 2.0–6.0 mmol/L, creatinine 266 mmol/L, normal range 80–120 mmol/L). Sputum was positive for AFB on direct smear.

Outcome

Quadruple therapy with antituberculous drugs and a full supportive regime of intravenous fluids was started, but the patient died 48 h after admission.

Comment

In white patients in the UK, disseminated and miliary tuberculosis tend to be more common in the elderly. Disease probably arises from a recrudescence of nascent infection which may have been present in the individual for many years. The elderly may be particularly susceptible to reactivation of remote infection, as cell-mediated immunity declines with age. The result is therefore more likely to be disseminated or miliary rather than pulmonary post-primary disease. Disseminated (sometimes called 'cryptic') disease is very difficult to diagnose, especially in the elderly. The symptoms are usually non-specific, the onset is insidious and multiple pathology is usual. The commonest symptoms are anorexia and weight loss. Pyrexia is common, and tuberculosis should be considered whenever an elderly patient presents with an unexplained fever. In retrospect it is difficult to see how the diagnosis could have been confirmed in this patient even if it had been considered at the time of her first admission. It is likely that a CT scan would have shown miliary seedlings in the lungs, which might have provided the diagnosis on transbronchial biopsy for histology and culture. However, in the presence of clear lung fields on plain chest X-ray such a series of investigations might have been difficult to justify. Alternatively, a liver or bone-marrow biopsy might have given the diagnosis.

As tuberculosis becomes less common among the white population in developed countries the index of suspicion has declined, and consequently the diagnosis is often made too late, as was the case with this patient. Diagnosis is often made post mortem. Tuberculin tests are frequently negative in elderly patients with disseminated disease.

Reference
Proudfoot, A.T. 1971: Cryptic disseminated tuberculosis. *British Journal of Hospital Medicine* **5**, 773–80.

SECTION 6H   GENITO-URINARY DISEASE

Case 74   A painful testicular swelling

Presenting complaint
A 52-year-old Pakistani man presented with a painful left testicular swelling.

History of presenting complaint
The patient had been aware of pain and discomfort in the left testicle for 4 weeks, and these symptoms had gradually increased. There had been no dysuria or haematuria. The patient had been living in the UK for 30 years, and his last return visit to Pakistan had been the previous year. There was no past medical history of note.

Examination
Examination revealed a tender lower left testis with some fluid in the scrotum.

Tests
An ultrasound scan showed a heterogeneous predominantly hypoechoic lesion in the anterior left testis which extended, possibly involving the scrotal wall. The kidneys were normal. The appearance was considered to resemble a testicular tumour.

Progress
The patient was listed for urgent orchidectomy. Three days prior to admission for this procedure there was discharge of pus from the left scrotum with a considerable reduction in pain. At operation the testicle was found to be attached to the skin where there was an abscess and multiple sinuses. An orchidectomy was performed as the testis had been largely destroyed. The specimen was opened on the table and was thought to show a tuberculous orchitis which was confirmed histologically. Samples were also sent for bacteriology, and these together with post-operative EMU samples were culture positive for fully sensitive M. tuberculosis. ESR was 22 mm/h, urea and electrolytes were normal and an intravenous pyelogram (IVP) showed no other evidence of urological tuberculosis. Treatment was commenced with Rifater, but a generalized rash developed after 4 days. Symptoms were controlled with terfenadine, but Rifater was stopped. After the rash had cleared, within a few days, rifampicin/isoniazid were given at standard dosage. Vomiting occurred but with normal liver function. The drugs were stopped and reintroduced gradually and sequentially with isoniazid first, and were then tolerated without difficulty. Since pyrazinamide could not be tolerated, and full sensitivity was later confirmed, treatment was given with rifampicin and isoniazid for 9 months in total.

Comment

Testicular or epididymal tuberculosis can simulate a tumour both clinically and ultrasonographically. Urological tuberculosis is the one form of tuberculosis which appears to be less common in immigrants from the Indian subcontinent living in the UK. A sinus had formed to the scrotum, and such scrofulodermatous involvement is seen in a proportion of renal or testicular tuberculosis cases. On finding epididymal or testicular tuberculosis, the rest of the urinary tract should be screened, as renal tuberculosis may coexist and have been the source of implantation, although haematogenous spread at primary infection is the more likely cause.

Reference

Gorse, R.J. and Belshe, R.B. 1985: Male genital tuberculosis: a review of the literature with illustrative case reports. *Review of Infectectious Diseases* **7**, 511–24.

Case 75   An unexpected finding

Presenting complaint
A 33-year-old white woman was admitted for routine laparoscopic sterilization.

History of presenting complaint
The patient had had two healthy deliveries and one miscarriage, and her two children were now aged 13 and 4 years. She had regular periods but had requested sterilization for contraceptive purposes. There was no other past medical history.

Examination
Preoperative general and gynaecological examination had been normal.

Tests
At laparoscopy the Fallopian tubes were seen to be thickened, so the procedure was converted to an open one. The right tube was clubbed and thickened at the fimbrial end, and a small focus of pus was found in the middle third. This was sent for standard culture and a partial salpingectomy was performed. There were adhesions around the left ovary which were dissected off and a left partial salpingectomy was carried out. Histology of both tubes showed large necrotizing palisaded granulomata in both tube walls with several small tuberculoid granulomata, with marked plasma cell and lymphocyte infiltration. The pus was negative for standard culture, but none was available for AFB culture.

Progress
On receipt of the histology the patient was referred to the chest service for management. Chest X-ray was normal, and there was a BCG vaccination scar. She had been a family contact of her stepfather, who had had smear- and culture-positive tuberculosis 5 years earlier. Treatment was given with Rifater for 2 months and then rifampicin/isoniazid for 4 months. The patient experienced facial flushing from the pyrazinamide in the first week of treatment, but there was no rash. Reassurance was given that the flushing was self-limiting, and this settled spontaneously.

Comment
Tuberculous salpingitis is sometimes found almost coincidentally during gynae-cological investigation, or it is found during investigation of primary or secondary infertility. This has to be differentiated from infertility due to intraperitoneal adhesions complicating peritoneal or intestinal tuberculosis which can also cause infertility without true tube involvement (fimbrial adhesions). In such cases there is seldom evidence of tuberculosis elsewhere in the body. Six-month short-course chemotherapy is adequate for these cases. If

the tubal damage is only moderate, a small percentage of cases regain fertility after treatment, but most depend on *in-vitro* fertilization (IVF) for further fertility if required.

Reference

Sutherland, A.M. 1985: Gynaecological tuberculosis: an analysis of a personal series of 710 cases. *Australian and New Zealand Journal of Obstetrics and Gynaecology* **25**, 203–7.

Case 76   Infertility

Presenting complaint
A 24-year-old Asian woman presented with primary infertility after 2.5 years of marriage.

History of presenting complaint
The patient had been living in the UK for 9 years, and had made one return visit to Pakistan when aged 14 years. Her periods had been regular, but she had not conceived after 2.5 years of unprotected intercourse. There were no constitutional features/symptoms and there was no past medical history.

Examination
Routine gynaecological and general examinations were normal.

Tests
The patient had an examination under anaesthetic, laparoscopy and dye test and dilatation and curettage (D and C). At laparoscopy both ovaries and the uterus were found to be normal. The tubes were both thickened with closed fimbrial ends. No dye was seen and no spill, suggesting bilateral cornual blockage. Endometrial curettings were sent for histology and culture. The endometrial histology showed scanty non-secretory endothelium containing multiple epithelioid granulomata with Langhans'-type giant cells, surrounded by lymphocytes, plasma cells and few polymorphs. These features strongly suggested tuberculous endometritis (Plate 76.1).

Progress
On receipt of the endometrial histology the patient was referred to the chest service for assessment and treatment. Chest X-ray was normal, haemoglobin was 12.0 g/dL normochromic but the ESR was 82 mm/h. The patient was started on rifampicin, isoniazid and pyrazinamide. After 5 weeks the endometrial curettings were culture positive for M. tuberculosis, which was later fully sensitive. The patient developed a generalized rash at 6 weeks. This settled with withdrawal of pyrazinamide. As fully sensitive organisms had been obtained, treatment with rifampicin/isoniazid was continued for a total of 9 months. D and C after completion of treatment showed normal endometrium, and cultures were negative. Because of the tubal damage, the patient was considered unsuitable for tubal surgery, and she was referred to an IVF programme.

Comment
Tubal and/or endometrial tuberculosis may be found in asymptomatic women who are being investigated for either primary or secondary infertility. The drug treatment of such cases, as with the patient described above, is best managed by the local thoracic physicians because of their knowledge of correct drug

regimens, dosages and side-effects. If the tuberculosis is purely endometrial, then fertility may be restored by eradicating the chronic endometritis. However, if there is coexisting tubal disease, whether or not this is amenable to tubal surgery or not will determine future fertility.

Case 77   The purulent postman

Presenting complaint
A 22-year-old Caucasian postman was referred because he had a history of a discharging sinus in the posterior loin area on the right for 5 years.

History of presenting complaint
At the age of 18 years the patient had suffered a non-specific illness during which he felt unwell and lost at least 10 kg in weight. He apparently made a good recovery after about 3 months, but it was as he was starting to feel better that he first noticed a painful swelling in the right loin posteriorly. A soft tender fluctuant lump measuring 5 cm by 5 cm was found 8 cm to the right of the mid-lumbar spine, which was incised, packed and drained. Approximately 1 year later the patient was admitted as an emergency case with an apparent recurrence of the abscess immediately to the right of the site of the healing scar from the first abscess. This was again excised, but no pus was found (Plate 77.1). What was thought to be a lipoma was removed. A further elective incision and drainage were performed 9 months later. The patient presented again after a further 9 months, now 3.5 years after the initial presentation, with a recurrence of the fluctuant swelling and a small discharging sinus. A sinogram showed a deep track to the psoas muscle. An IVP showed punctate calcification in the right kidney, which was confirmed by CT scan (Fig. 77.1). At this time cultures for AAFB were sent from the wound and EMU samples, but all remained negative.

Progress
After referral from general surgery to the urology department, the patient was referred on to the chest physician, 5 years after his initial presentation. Triple antituberculosis therapy in the form of Rifater (isoniazid, rifampicin and pyrazinamide) was started. Pyrazinamide was stopped after 2 months and the other medication was continued for a total of 6 months. During the time on treatment the scar area healed and the sinus stopped discharging.

Six months after treatment was stopped, the swelling recurred and the sinus again began to discharge. Repeated cultures for AFB, other bacteria and fungi were negative. Triple therapy was again started, reducing to isoniazid and rifampicin at 2 months. Eight months later, and while the patient was on these two drugs, the sinus again began to discharge. Ethambutol, ciprofloxacin and prednisolone (0.5 mg/kg) were added. Little change was seen over the next 6 months, and the abscess continued to swell and discharge intermittently. Prednisolone was stopped after 6 months.

At 8 months after the two additional drugs were given and 14 months after the start of the second course of treatment, the sinus had not discharged for 2 months. After a further 6 months, and 20 months after the start of the second

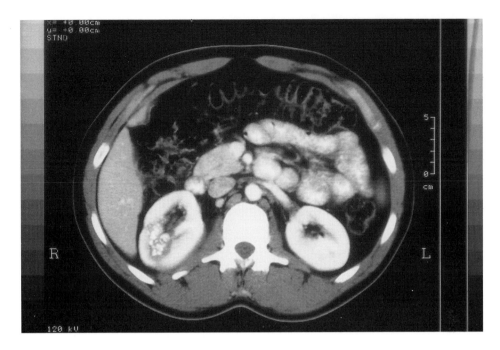

Fig. 77.1

course, there had been no further discharge and the scar appeared to be well healed. This was 7 years after the initial presentation.

Comment

Although there is no bacterial or histological proof of tuberculosis, this case has all the hallmarks of a chronic tuberculous abscess, perhaps originating in the kidney but then tracking posteriorly to form a chronic sinus in the back. It was unfortunate that no specimens for bacteriology or histology appear to have been available from the first operation. The diagnosis of tuberculosis does not appear to have been considered until 4 years after the initial presentation. The main problem in this case arises from the apparent relapse after initial treatment, and the relapse for a second time while apparently on adequate therapy.

Management was further compounded by the inability to grow organisms from the pus and therefore to obtain sensitivities. The cause of the two relapses was probably lack of compliance, although the possibility of an immunological reaction with sterile swelling of the abscess was considered, which is why prednisolone as well as two new drugs were added to the regimen.

The patient was clinically well during all this time, and at no point could the disease be said to be life-threatening, so the addition of three second-line drugs did not appear to be warranted. Treatment was stopped after 2 years. A year later, the disease had not recurred.

Reference

Humphries, M.J. and Lam, W.K. 1998: Non-respiratory tuberculosis. In Davies, P.D.O. (ed.), *Clinical tuberculosis*. London: Chapman and Hall, 175–204.

SECTION 61   ABDOMINAL DISEASE

Case 78   Abdominal pains

Presenting complaint
A 20-year-old Indian woman presented with a history of 14 days of colicky right iliac fossa pain.

History of presenting complaint
The patient was born in the UK, and had made a single visit to India 7 years previously. She gave a history of right iliac fossa pain occurring over a 3- to 4-year period. The pain would be present for several weeks at a time but there would be intervals of up to a few months without symptoms. For 14 days the pain had been worse, severe and colicky in nature, and the patient had been vomiting for 1 day. She stated that no weight loss had occurred.

Past medical history
The patient had been investigated for this pain about 2 years earlier but blood tests, gastroscopy and abdominal ultrasound had been normal.

Examination
The patient was afebrile, and the abdomen showed a mass in the right iliac fossa with increased bowel sounds.

Tests
An ultrasound scan of the abdomen showed thickened bowel in the region of the terminal ileum and caecum. Chest X-ray was normal. Haemoglobin was 8.0 g/dL with an MCV of 55.9 fL and a low ferritin concentration at 6.0 U/L (normal range 15–100 U/L). ESR was 26 mm/h, CRP was 78 (normal range 0–6) and serum albumen was low at 25 g/L. The tuberculin test was positive (Heaf grade 3). Barium follow-through showed irregular stricturing extending from the terminal ileum to the caecum and proximal ascending colon, with mucosal nodularity and ulceration with one or two areas of fissuring (Fig. 78.1). The appearances were thought to be consistent with Crohn's disease, but tuberculosis was given as a differential diagnosis.

Progress
Because of continuing pain and features suggestive of subacute intestinal obstruction, a laparotomy was performed. An inflammatory mass involving the distal 10 cm of ileum, the caecum and ascending colon was found adherent to the posterior abdominal wall. This was thought to be a Crohn's mass. It was

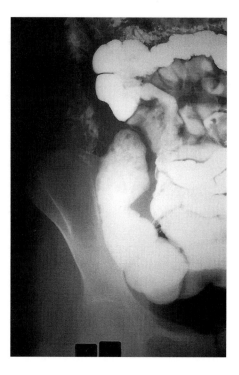

Fig. 78.1

mobilized and a standard right hemicolectomy was performed. Histology showed multiple granulomata in all levels of the bowel wall and in the mesenteric glands. In some areas they coalesced to give caseation, and AFB were seen on ZN staining in both lymph nodes and bowel wall. Triple therapy as a combination tablet plus ethambutol (15 mg/kg) was given for 2 months, followed by rifampicin/isoniazid as combination therapy for a further 4 months. The haemoglobin, CRP and albumen levels returned to normal and the patient gained 9.5 kg during the treatment period.

Comment

Tuberculous enteritis cannot be differentiated from inflammatory bowel disease either radiologically or macroscopically. In ethnic-minority patients tuberculosis is much more common than Crohn's disease, and in white patients inflammatory bowel disease is much more common than tuberculosis. Samples should always be taken for culture for AFB at operation because macroscopically the two conditions cannot be separated reliably. One-third of abdominal tuberculosis cases have a short acute presentation simulating an appendicitis, and one-third present with a chronic illness lasting months or even years (as in this case) with abdominal colicky pain which may be intermittent. The remainder present with either diffuse 'plastic peritonitis' (see Case 79) or ascites (see Case 80).

Reference

Klimach, O.E. and Ormerod, L.P. 1985: Gastrointestinal tuberculosis: a retrospective review of 109 cases in a district general hospital. *Quarterly Journal of Medicine* **56**, 569–78.

Case 79   Marked weight loss

Presenting complaint

A 15-year-old Indian girl was seen with abdominal pain and weight loss of over 20 kg.

History of presenting complaint

The patient had an 8-month history of intermittent central abdominal pain, and had lost over 20 kg in the same period of time. She had developed secondary amenorrhoea, and had had intermittent vomiting for 2 months. She was born in the UK and had made one visit to India 8 years earlier.

Examination

There was obvious weight loss (total body weight 36 kg), but there were no focal signs in the abdomen and no ascites.

Tests

Ultrasound scan of the abdomen showed normal liver and spleen, no ascites, but possible loops of bowel in the left iliac fossa. ESR was in the range 23–45 mm/h. Haemoglobin was 11.8 g/dL, with a serum albumen concentration of 31 g/L and a globulin level of 47 g/L. A barium meal showed possible deformity in the lesser curve, but gastroscopy showed no ulcer, bile-stained fluid and a positive helicobacter-like organism (HLO) result. HLO eradication therapy made no difference to the patient's symptoms, and a later abdominal X-ray suggested subacute intestinal obstruction. Laparotomy was performed, during which an intense plastic peritonitis was encountered. There were multiple peritoneal nodules, the omentum was thickened and the small bowel loops were all matted together. The peritonitis was so intense that only an omental biopsy could be safely carried out.

Progress

The surgeon who performed the operation recognized this case as tuberculous peritonitis, and asked the thoracic physician to come to theatre to begin management. A feeding line was inserted under the anaesthetic, and treatment with rifampicin (450 mg), isoniazid (300 mg) IV, streptomycin 0.75 g IM daily and dexamethasone 4 mg tds IV was started with full parenteral nutrition. Ceftriaxone and flagyl were also given for 7 days to cover wound infection and bowel sepsis. After 2 weeks the patient was able to take fluids, and the treatment was changed to Rifater 4 tablets and streptomycin was stopped. After 4 weeks the patient developed a swinging fever with normal liver function. An abdominal ultrasound scan showed a pelvic abscess which was drained per rectum (500 mL) and found to be coliform. Omental cultures confirmed M. tuberculosis, and histology also showed granulomata with caseation and scattered AFB. The patient required 2 months of hospitalization as an in-patient, gaining

8 kg. Treatment with rifampicin/isoniazid continued for a further 4 months, and her weight at the end of treatment was 58.8 kg. There was no recurrence of tuberculosis on follow-up, but several years later she was investigated for infertility due to her abdominal disease.

Comment

In the above case weight loss and systemic symptoms predominated. There was no change in bowel habit and no ascites. Laparoscopy is normally the investigation of choice, but if intense plastic peritonitis is suspected, laparotomy may be safer, with a lower likelihood of bowel perforation. Parenteral nutrition may be needed together with antituberculosis drugs and corticosteroids to help to reduce the inflammatory response. Antituberculosis therapy may also need to be given intravenously or by IM injection until absorption from the bowel is possible. Ten per cent of females with abdominal tuberculosis suffer from infertility after the illness due to peritoneal adhesions.

Case 80   Postpartum fever

Presenting complaint
A 38-year-old Asian woman who had just delivered her fifth child was seen with fever 6 weeks post delivery.

History of presenting complaint
The patient had lived in the UK for 30 years and had made a single visit to Pakistan 7 years earlier. Since her delivery she had experienced some sweats and fever at night, and she felt that her abdomen had not gone down as quickly after delivery as in her previous pregnancies.

Past medical history
The patient had previously been investigated for right upper quadrant pain, with gallstones found on ultrasound, but hepatitis screening had been negative for hepatitis B and C.

Examination
The patient showed fever to 38.5°C and moderate abdominal distension.

Tests
Chest X-ray was normal, ESR was 72 mm/h, blood cultures were negative and the globulin level was raised at 38 g/L. A repeat abdominal ultrasound scan showed gallstones, a normal liver and bile ducts, but moderate ascites. Ascitic tap showed an exudate (protein content 67 g/L) which was found to contain many lymphocytes on cytology. Some ascitic fluid was sent for tuberculosis culture.

Progress
A laparoscopy was performed during which 1600 mL of ascitic fluid were removed, and the surface of the bowel, the omentum and the peritoneum were found to be studded with tubercles. Biopsy of the omental nodules confirmed caseating granulomata, and omental biopsy and ascitic fluid were later positive for M. *tuberculosis* on culture. The organism was fully sensitive. After the laparoscopy triple therapy was started pending histological confirmation. The fever settled in 4 days. Standard 6-month short-course chemotherapy was given which was uncomplicated. The ascites resolved completely, and all blood tests returned to normal. Secondary infertility occurred after treatment.

Comment
Tuberculous ascites, in common with other serous membrane tuberculosis, produces a lymphocyte-rich exudate, and this feature alone should raise a high index of suspicion. In areas with poor health provision, treatment may have to be given on suspicion on the basis of these data. Laparoscopy is the investigation

of choice in such cases, as biopsies for histology and culture can be taken. If the ultrasound scan suggests that loops of bowel may be adherent to the anterior abdominal wall, insertion of the Verres needle must be done with care in order to reduce the risk of bowel perforation. The fluid resolves on treatment, together with constitutional symptoms. Infertility (either primary or secondary) is reported in 10 per cent of females treated for abdominal tuberculosis, and is thought to be due to intra-abdominal adhesions involving the ovary and/or fimbria of the Fallopian tubes.

Reference
Manohar, A., Simjee, A.E. and Haffejee A.A. 1990: Symptoms and investigative findings in 145 patients with tuberculous peritonitis diagnosed by peritoneoscopy and biopsy over a five-year period. *Gut* **31**, 1130–2.

Case 81   Profound weight loss

Presenting complaint
A 29-year-old Pakistani man presented with weight loss of 25 kg over 6 months.

History of presenting complaint
The patient had lived in the UK for 15 years, and had stayed in Pakistan for 6 months 2 years earlier. He gave a history of weight loss, poor appetite and evening fever. He also stated that if he ate food it appeared per rectum about 1 h later. There had been a little blood in his stools and he had experienced intermittent vomiting. There was no past medical history of note.

Examination
The patient was thin (60 kg) with no ascites or palpable abdominal masses.

Tests
Haemoglobin was 9.7 g/dL, MCV was 64 fL, ESR was 70 mm/h and albumen was 35 g/L. Ferritin was normal and haemoglobin electrophoresis showed increased HbA2 (beta-thalassaemia minor). Chest X-ray showed right hilar lymph-adenopathy and some right lower zone infiltration (Fig. 81.1). Two sputum

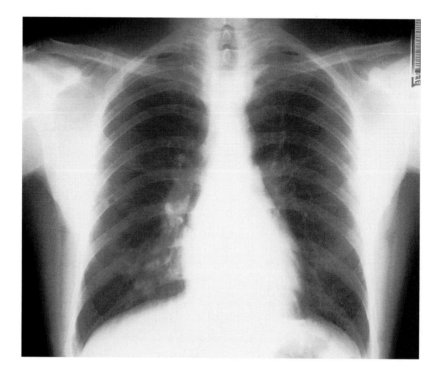

Fig. 81.1

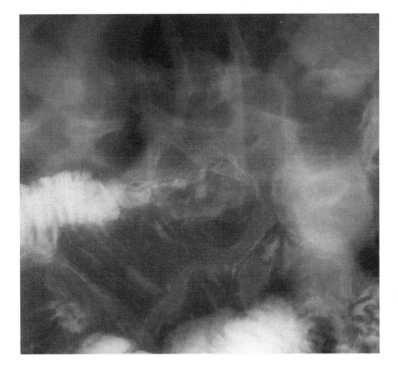

Fig. 81.2

samples were negative on microscopy for AFB. Barium follow-through showed barium in the colon by 40 min and some localized jejunal stenosis (Fig. 81.2). Treatment with Rifater and ethambutol was started.

Progress

Despite treatment the patient continued to vomit and lose weight. Plain X-rays showed no true intestinal obstruction and liver function was normal. Parenteral nutrition and intravenous rifampicin/isoniazid were started but there was no improvement. A laparotomy was performed which showed widespread peritoneal nodules and adhesions, obstruction at the ileo-caecal valve and a jejunal obstruction. Jejunal and ileo-ascending colon anastomoses were performed after the obstructing bowel had been resected. Histology confirmed tuberculous strictures. Intravenous feeding and treatment continued until intestinal motility was resumed, and the patient was then switched back to oral therapy. Sputum was culture positive for fully sensitive M. *tuberculosis*. The patient weighed 53 kg at the nadir. Treatment was given for 2 months with Rifater and ethambutol after surgery, and then rifampicin/isoniazid were given for a further 4 months. The patient weighed 81 kg at the end of treatment.

Comment

An ileocolic fistula was suspected from the history but was not confirmed at barium follow-through. Tuberculosis was the initial diagnosis before the chest X-ray showed compatible changes. Abdominal tuberculosis can mimic Crohn's disease on barium, with 'skip' lesions, Kantor's string sign of ileo-caecal narrowing, and even fistulae. Tuberculous masses in the ileo-caecal area or in the colon can simulate carcinoma. If there is no intestinal obstruction, laparoscopy is the investigation of choice. Resection is only required if there is mechanical obstruction, but multiple levels can be involved. Six-month short-course chemotherapy gives good results.

Case 82 Perianal mass and bleeding

Presenting complaint
A frail 92-year-old Asian woman presented with a history of rectal bleeding for 3 weeks.

History of presenting complaint
The patient had had a surgical haemorrhoidectomy 3 years earlier. She reported a history of some alteration of bowel habit and occasional faecal incontinence for 6 months, with infrequent blood, but more regular rectal bleeding for 3 weeks.

Past medical history
Haemorrhoidectomy had been performed 3 years earlier when sigmoidoscopy was otherwise normal to 20 cm.

Examination
The patient was thin and cachectic (36 kg). There was an ulcerated mass posteriorly at the anal margin (Plates 82.1 and 82.2).

Tests
Haemoglobin was 11.0 g/dL and ESR was 46 mm/h. An examination under anaesthetic (EUA) and sigmoidoscopy were performed. The ulcerated mass at the 7 o'clock position was considered clinically to be a carcinoma, but sigmoidoscopy showed the lesion to extend 10 cm upwards. Biopsies were taken from the edge of the lesion. The biopsies showed multiple granulomata with Langhans' cells and areas of central necrosis. There was also large bowel mucosa and some squamous epithelium derived from the anal canal. A few AFB were present on ZN staining.

Progress
The surgeons, who had been convinced clinically that this was an anal carcinoma, referred the patient to the chest service. She had no respiratory symptoms, but chest X-ray showed old calcified disease in the right upper zone. She was treated with Rifater; ethambutol was not given as she had senile cataracts and poor vision. Rifater was given for 2 months, and then rifampicin/isoniazid for a further 4 months as combination therapy, all supervised by the patient's family. The lesion resolved over 4 months, leaving only a small scar at the completion of treatment.

Comment
Tuberculosis can simulate carcinoma in the large bowel or at the anal margin. There was no associated abscess or sinus in this case. Biopsies from apparently malignant-looking lesions can sometimes give surprises! What looked like a

surgically untreatable case was cured medically. The drug treatment of all non-respiratory tuberculosis should be supervised only by physicians who are experienced in tuberculosis management (normally a thoracic physician). Despite her advanced age, the patient had no drug-related side-effects, but was given pyridoxine 10 mg/day.

Reference
Klimach, O.E. and Ormerod, L.P. 1985: Gastrointestinal tuberculosis: a retrospective review of 109 cases in a district general hospital. *Quarterly Journal of Medicine* **56**, 569–78.

Cross reference
Chapter 11, Altered diagnosis

Case 83   An elderly Mexican man with weight loss and fever

Presenting complaint
A 71-year-old Mexican man presented with weight loss of 28 kg and recent fever.

History of presenting complaint
The patient had experienced insidious weight loss and anorexia over 12 months. He had had a gastroscopy some months earlier when mild gastritis was found, and he had been taking ranitidine since then. Two weeks prior to presentation he had developed daily fever and sweats. He denied cough, breathlessness or sputum production.

Past medical history
The patient had had transurethral resection of the prostate 2 years earlier.

Examination
Marked weight loss was apparent, and the patient was febrile at 38.9°C. There was generalized 1- to 2-cm lymph-node enlargement of the posterior and anterior cervical, supraclavicular, axillary and inguinal glands bilaterally. The liver was palpable 2 cm below the costal margin, and was smooth but mildly tender.

Tests
Chest X-ray was normal. ESR was 110 mm/h. Sodium was 125 mmol/L, alkaline phosphatase was 220 IU/mL, and bilirubin and hepatic transaminases were normal. The tuberculin test (Mantoux) was negative. A CT of the abdomen demonstrated diffuse enlargement of the retroperitoneal and mesenteric nodes (Fig. 83.1) and a complex mass involving the left lobe of the liver (Fig. 83.2). There were no pulmonary nodules or infiltrates on the CT scan. A CT-guided liver biopsy into the left lobe showed chronic inflammation without granuloma formation, and special stains for mycobacteria were negative. During the tests the patient continued to be febrile up to 40.0°C. A lymph-node biopsy of a cervical gland was performed, which showed necrotizing granulomata with AFB.

Progress
Treatment with rifampicin, isoniazid, pyrazinamide and ethambutol was started after the cervical histology. Within 4 days the patient felt better and was afebrile. Drug-susceptible M. *tuberculosis* was grown from the lymph-node biopsy. The patient was discharged from hospital and was subsequently treated with a DOT delivered to his home twice weekly. He regained 23 kg before he completed his 6-month treatment. A repeat CT scan of the abdomen showed resolution of the hepatic abnormalities and enlarged intra-abdominal nodes.

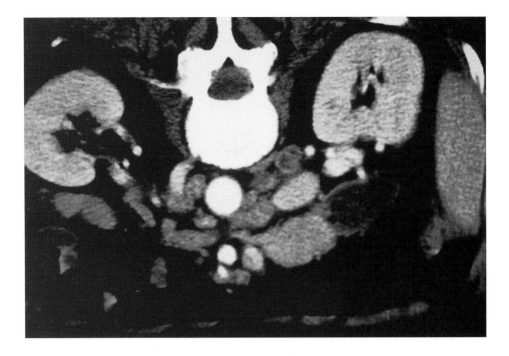

Fig. 83.1

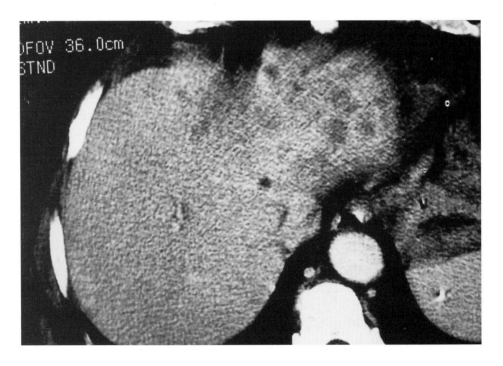

Fig. 83.2

Comment

The usual presentation of tuberculous lymphadenopathy is the enlargement of a single or multiple nodes in a single anatomical chain. Diffuse adenopathy, as in this case, is uncommon, being described in only 3 per cent of nodal cases. It is more common in individuals with miliary disease, but there was no evidence of miliary involvement even on sensitive CT scan. Essentially the patient had 'cryptic disseminated' or 'late generalized' tuberculosis in which, due to the lack of classical miliary involvement, the diagnosis is often delayed and mortality is high. The CT appearance of the liver suggested a malignant pathology, and tuberculosis was not considered in the radiological differential diagnosis. Hepatic involvement is very common in disseminated tuberculosis, but is usually a diffuse granulomatous infiltration rather than a focal mass. However, this patient's pattern of liver involvement is well documented as either 'tuberculous pseudotumour' or 'macronodular hepatic tuberculosis'.

References

Achem, S.R., Kolts, B.E., Grisnik, J. et al. 1992: Pseudotumoral hepatic tuberculosis: atypical presentation and comprehensive review of the literature. Journal of Clinical Gastroenterology 14, 72–7.

Kent, D.C. 1987: Tuberculous lymphadenitis: not a localised disease process. American Journal of Medical Sciences 1967, 866–73.

Cross reference

Chapter 6, Section 6G, Miliary disease

SECTION 6J LYMPH-NODE DISEASE

Case 84 The foreign student

Presenting complaint
A 25-year-old Malaysian student was referred with a 6-week history of cervical lymphadenopathy.

History of presenting complaint
The lymphadenopathy had been present for 6 weeks, was more marked on the left, and had been relatively painless. There had been no discharge.

Previous medical history
There was a possible history of BCG vaccination at the age 12 years.

Examination
There were some small glands in the right neck at 1–2 cm, but there were larger 3-cm nodes in the left neck. There was no other lymphadenopathy or hepatosplenomegaly.

Tests
Chest X-ray showed no mediastinal glands. Haemoglobin was 13.7 g/dL, ESR was 74 mm/h and the tuberculin test was strongly positive (Heaf 3). As the patient was about to return to Malaysia for the summer vacation he was advised to have a lymph-node biopsy for histology and tuberculosis culture.

Progress
The patient returned to the UK after his summer vacation having had a gland biopsy which confirmed tuberculosis histologically, but no cultures had been collected. He had been on treatment with rifampicin (600 mg), isoniazid (300 mg), pyrazinamide (1500 mg) and streptomycin (1.0 g) daily for 8 weeks (for body weight 59.5 kg). Pyrazinamide and streptomycin were stopped, and treatment was continued with rifampicin/isoniazid. After a further 2 months, a new small fluctuant left cervical gland developed as well as discharging sinuses at the biopsy site. Pus was aspirated from the fluctuant gland but was culture negative. Rifampicin/isoniazid were continued and, on receipt of negative cultures, prednisolone (25 mg/day) was added. There was a slow improvement in the sinuses and the gland on the left. A new 3-cm gland then appeared on the right, but the sinuses on the left healed. This gland was biopsied for culture and was again negative.

   The glands on both sides then slowly resolved and steroids were tailed off over a 2-month period. Treatment with rifampicin/isoniazid was given for a total of 9 months.

Comment

The development of new glands, enlargement of existing glands and the development of sinuses occur in about 20 per cent of cases of lymph-node tuberculosis in controlled trials. These phenomena can also occur after drug treatment has finished, and do not of themselves suggest relapse. The difficulty in this case was that there was no bacteriology, and since primary drug resistance occurs in approximately 5 per cent of cases in ethnic-minority groups, the possibility of failure due to drug resistance could not be excluded. Once negative cultures had been received, treatment with corticosteroids to reduce the excessive immune response which is thought to lead to such phenomena was started. Six-month short-course chemotherapy has been shown to be just as effective as longer treatment. In this case a longer treatment was used because of the lack of culture and drug-resistance data. Surgeons dealing with a suspected tuberculous gland, or any persistent gland in an ethnic-minority patient, should routinely send half of the gland in a *dry* pot for tuberculosis culture. The persistence of lymphadenopathy at the end of treatment, and particularly the development of lymph-node enlargement or new lymphadenopathy during or after treatment, causes concern to physicians who are not experienced in treating lymph-node disease. These concerns might lead to the unnecessary extension of treatment or the reintroduction of treatment for 'relapse'. Such events occur in up to 20 per cent of cases during treatment and in up to 15 per cent of cases after treatment. These nodes, if biopsied, are usually negative on culture, and although clinical 'relapse' may be diagnosed, they are bacteriologically sterile. It is likely that such phenomena are immunologically related, being due to hypersensitivity to tuberculoprotein, perhaps from disrupted macrophages, and that they do not indicate an unfavourable outcome.

References

British Thoracic Society Research Committee. 1992: Six-months versus nine-months chemotherapy for tuberculosis of lymph nodes: preliminary results. *Respiratory Medicine* **83**, 15–19.

British Thoracic Society Research Committee. 1993: Six-months versus nine-months chemotherapy for tuberculosis of lymph nodes: final results. *Respiratory Medicine* **87**, 621–3.

Case 85   Massive lymphadenopathy

Presenting complaint
A 48-year-old Pakistani man presented with rapidly developing lymphadeno-pathy in the right neck.

History of presenting complaint
The patient had lived in the UK for over 20 years. Over 3 to 4 weeks he had developed painful right cervical lymphadenopathy which had enlarged rapidly. He had not lost weight, and there was no other lymphadenopathy. He had had an anterior myocardial infarction at the age of 46 years.

Examination
There was extensive firm non-fluctuant lymphadenopathy extending in a solid mass from the angle of the jaw down to the clavicle. There was no erythema and no lymphadenopathy in the left neck, either axilla or the groin. There was also no hepatosplenomegaly.

Tests
Chest X-ray was normal. Haemoglobin was 16.1 g/dL, WCC was 6.2×10^6/mL, and ESR was 10 mm/h. Ultrasound examination showed the neck mass to consist of multiple well-defined nodular masses. A gland biopsy of the neck mass showed dual pathology. In some areas the excised node was replaced by a high-grade non-Hodgkin lymphoma (Plate 85.1) and in other areas by caseous granulomatous material with AFB visualized (Plate 85.2). Although the gland had been considered to be macroscopically malignant, a sample had been routinely sent for tuberculosis culture.

Progress
A CT scan of the chest and abdomen for staging showed some abdominal para-aortic nodes, but none in the pelvis or chest. The liver and spleen were normal. Bone marrow and trephine were also normal. For the lymphoma, combination therapy including bleomycin was given, with radiotherapy to the right neck nodal mass. Treatment for tuberculosis was given concurrently with Rifater 6 tablets (for body weight 73 kg), and a regular anti-emetic because of the cyclical chemotherapy. Positive cultures for M. tuberculosis were obtained from the gland biopsy that were fully sensitive to first-line drugs. After 2 months the patient was switched from Rifater to Rifinah 300 (2 tablets) for a further 4 months. The lymphoma went into remission with six cycles of chemotherapy. The patient died of heart failure 3 years later without recurrence of either lymphoma or tuberculosis.

Comment
In this case malignancy rather than tuberculosis was suspected because of the very rapid enlargement of the glands without fluctuation. However, the surgeon

routinely sent part of the gland for tuberculosis culture in ethnic-minority groups, irrespective of his clinical diagnosis. The dual pathology was a surprise, but each element was treated individually. Malignancy, particularly lymphoma, is a risk factor for tuberculosis. This was added to the increased risk of an ethnic-minority group with rates 25 times those found among the white ethnic group. It was interesting that the disease coexisted in the same gland, suggesting but not proving that the breakdown of local immune surveillance caused the reactivation disease. Standard 6-month short-course chemotherapy was given, and gave a cure despite concurrent chemotherapy and radiotherapy. Such 6-month regimens have been shown to perform just as well as 9-month regimens in lymph-node tuberculosis.

SECTION 6K   SKIN TUBERCULOSIS

Case 86   A painful sternum

Presenting complaint
A 62-year-old Asian man presented with a discharging sinus over the mid-sternum.

History of presenting complaint
The patient had been living in the UK for 5 years. He had been aware of discomfort in the central sternum for 2 months, which he described as 'like a punch'. The area had then reddened, discharged and continued to discharge. He had lost 2 or 3 kg but had no other constitutional features and no cough or sputum. There was no past medical history of note.

Examination
This showed a discharging sinus over the mid-sternum (Plate 86.1). There were no signs in the chest and no neck glands were palpable.

Tests
Postero-anterior (PA) chest X-ray showed some calcification in the paratracheal glands but no enlargement, and the lung fields were clear. Lateral chest X-ray showed a pathological fracture of the sternum. Haemoglobin was 11.9 g/dL normochromic with an ESR of 38 mm/h. Biopsy from the skin edge showed multiple granulomata with Langhans' giant cells. The tuberculin test was strongly positive. Material from the sinus was sent for tuberculosis culture, but was negative on direct microscopy.

Progress
A clinical diagnosis of scrofuloderma was made, and treatment with rifampicin, isoniazid, pyrazinamide and ethambutol was commenced immediately after the biopsy and samples had been taken. The lesion healed slowly and required packing with a wick to prevent skin closure before the base had healed. M. tuberculosis grew from the pre-treatment samples at 5 weeks, and full sensitivity was confirmed. Pyrazinamide and ethambutol were stopped at 8 weeks, and rifampicin and isoniazid were continued for a further 4 months. Skin healing had occurred by 2 months, and sternal bony union by 4 months. There was no recurrence during a 15-month follow-up.

Comment
Scrofuloderma is tuberculous skin involvement due to tuberculosis of a deeper structure eroding through on to the skin and discharging. This is a particular complication of lymph-node disease, genito-urinary disease and, as in this case,

bony disease. In most developed countries it is the commonest cause of skin tuberculosis. In addition to standard short-course chemotherapy, a deep sinus may need to be packed to allow healing from the base. If skin closure occurs leaving a potential space below, secondary infection can occur.

References

Beyt, B.E., Ortbals, D.W., Santa Crus, D.J. *et al.* 1981: Cutaneous mycobacteriosis: analysis of 34 cases with a new classification of disease. *Medicine* **60**, 95–109.

Yates, V.M. and Ormerod, L.P. 1997: Cutaneous tuberculosis in Blackburn District (UK): a 15-year prospective series 1981–95. *British Journal of Dermatology* **136**, 483–9.

Case 87 A few funny patches

Presenting complaint
A 52-year-old Indian man was seen with three skin patches.

History of presenting complaint
Over 2 to 3 months the patient had developed three separate painless violaceous skin patches, one on the left pinna, one on the right upper arm and one on the left flank, the latter two measuring 3 × 4 cm. These patches had been non-tender and non-itchy, and had gradually enlarged. They were slightly raised, and the lesion on the pinna was a little scaly.

Previous medical history
The patient had had pulmonary tuberculosis in India 25 years previously. At that time he was treated with streptomycin, isoniazid and para-aminosalicylic acid (PAS), but he was unsure of the duration of therapy.

Examination
There was a violaceous rash over the left pinna, with slight scaling (Plate 87.1), and two other lesions on the right upper arm and left flank. There were no signs in the chest, no lymphadenopathy and no hepatosplenomegaly.

Tests
Chest X-ray showed a little calcified scarring at the left apex. The patient had no sputum to test and bronchoscopy was not performed. A tuberculin test was not performed either in view of the previous history of tuberculosis. The lesion on the flank was biopsied and showed multiple granulomata in the dermis extending into the epidermis. A clinical and histological diagnosis of lupus vulgaris was made. No AFB were seen on microscopy, and a piece of skin was sent for culture.

Progress
Treatment with rifampicin, isoniazid, pyrazinamide and ethambutol was started after the biopsy. The lesions regressed over 8 weeks, and virtually normal skin was restored. Pyrazinamide and ethambutol were stopped after 8 weeks. Cultures from the skin were negative. Treatment with rifampicin/isoniazid was continued for a further 7 months because of the previous history of tuberculosis and lack of sensitivity data. No recurrence was seen during a 15-month follow-up.

Comment
Lupus vulgaris can often be diagnosed clinically and represents true skin infection in a tuberculin-sensitized host. Granulomata in the skin and the presence of AFB on biopsy should always raise the possibility of a different mycobacterial disease caused by M. leprae. A check for anaesthesia around the

lesion and related peripheral nerve thickening should be made. Lupus vulgaris responds rapidly to standard short-course chemotherapy. A longer treatment was given here because of the patient's previous history.

Reference
Rameshh, V., Misra, R.S., Saxena, U. *et al.* 1991: Comparative efficacy of drug regimens in skin tuberculosis. *Clinical and Experimental Dermatology* **16**, 106–9.

Case 88 Recurrent skin lesions

Presenting complaint
A 34-year-old East African Asian woman presented with a history of recurrent skin lesions.

History of presenting complaint
Over a 5-year period the patient had had crops of skin lesions on the calves which looked somewhat like bruises, were painful but not itchy, and were associated with some fever. The lesions had settled over 1 or 2 months, each time without medical intervention. There were no systemic features.

Past medical history
The patient had been seen about 8 years earlier as a contact of a family case of tuberculosis. At that time she had a normal X-ray but a strongly positive Mantoux (to 1 TU).

Examination
General examination was normal. There were lesions up to 5 cm in diameter on the calves which were very suggestive of a panniculitis (Plate 88.1).

Tests
Chest X-ray was normal. Haemoglobin was 13.8 g/dL normochromic and ESR was 18 mm/h. A biopsy of one of the lesions showed panniculitis in the subcutaneous fat, with the inflammatory cells being lymphocytes and epithelioid histiocytes, and an occasional Langhans' giant cell was present. The appearances were thought to be very suggestive of tuberculous panniculitis or erythema induratum (Bazin's disease). Serology for syphilis was negative.

Progress
Treatment with rifampicin, isoniazid and pyrazinamide was given for 2 months, and the lesions resolved rapidly. Rifampicin and isoniazid were continued for a further 4 months. There was no recurrence of the lesions over an 18-month follow-up period.

Comment
The diagnosis of the tuberculides, of which panniculitis and Bazin's disease are examples, depends on clinical suspicion and histology (which is consistent), supported by a positive tuberculin test. Primary skin tuberculosis is paucibacillary, with culture confirmation being rare. Mycobacterium-tuberculosis-complex DNA has been identified by polymerase chain reaction in routinely fixed samples in lupus vulgaris and in all other forms of skin tuberculosis (see below). This method has recently been compared to culture of these skin lesions and has been shown to give a higher diagnostic yield. This may have applications in

developed countries, but in resource-poor countries a trial of treatment may be all that is available.

References

Margall, N., Baselga, E., Coll, P. *et al.* 1996: Detection of Mycobacterium tuberculosis complex DNA by the polymerase chain reaction for the rapid diagnosis of cutaneous tuberculosis. *British Journal of Dermatology* **135**, 231–6.

Penney, S.N.S., Leonarch, C.L., Cock, S. *et al.* 1993: Identification of Mycobacterium tuberculosis DNA in 5 different types of cutaneous lesions by the polymerase chain reaction. *Archives of Dermatology* **129**, 1594–8.

Case 89   More funny lumps

Presenting complaint
A 16-year-old Asian girl was seen with widespread papular lesions on both thighs and shins.

History of presenting complaint
The patient was born in the UK but had made one visit to India at age 5 years. She had developed multiple lesions on both thighs and shins which were itchy, papular and lichenified but non-flexural. A few of these had developed into very superficial ulcers. There was no past medical history.

Examination
There were multiple lesions on both anterior thighs and shins (Plate 89.1). There was no nerve thickening and no anaesthesia. General examination was normal.

Tests
Chest X-ray was normal. Haemoglobin was 11.3 g/dL with an MCV of 69.3 fL. Haemoglobin electrophoresis showed beta-thalassaemia minor. Liver function was normal and the tuberculin test was strongly positive. Biopsy of one of the lesions which had ulcerated showed granulomata and fibrinoid necrosis at the base of the ulcer. There were perivascular infiltrates of plasma cells and lymphocytes. The dermis contained several follicular aggregates of epithelioid cells and a few Langhans' giant cells.

Progress
A form of cutaneous tuberculosis, namely lichen scrofulosum, was suspected. The skin biopsy together with the tuberculin test were considered to be sufficient for a trial of treatment. Rifampicin, isoniazid and pyrazinamide were given for 2 months, with rifampicin/isoniazid for a further 4 months. The lesions cleared substantially during the first 3 months of treatment and did not recur in a follow-up period of over 18 months.

Comment
This is another form of cutaneous tuberculosis which is less common than erythema induratum and lupus vulgaris. Mycobacterial DNA has also been demonstrated in such cases. Clinical suspicion supported by a strongly positive tuberculin test and consistent histology constitute sufficient grounds for a therapeutic trial of antituberculosis therapy.

Reference
Penney, S.N.S., Leonarch, C.L., Cock, S. et al. 1993: Identification of Mycobacterium tuberculosis DNA in 5 different cutaneous lesions by the polymerase chain reaction. Archives of Dermatology 129, 1594–8.

Childhood disease

Case 90   A newly arrived Pakistani boy

Presenting complaint
A 5-year-old asymptomatic Pakistani boy was seen for new-immigrant screening.

History of presenting complaint
The patient had been born of Pakistani parents in the UK and had had a BCG vaccination at birth. He had spent 3 years (from ages 2 to 5 years) in Pakistan and was screened after returning to the UK because he had stayed in a high-prevalence country (as defined by an annual incidence of 40 in 100 000 or greater). His mother said that he was not eating well but otherwise he had no symptoms.

Past medical history
The patient had had normal childhood vaccinations but no known contact with tuberculosis.

Examination
The patient was afebrile, there were no physical signs, and he weighed 22 kg.

Tests
The tuberculin test was strongly positive (Heaf 4), which was not consistent with the child's BCG history. Chest X-ray was performed, which showed right paratracheal lymphadenopathy (Fig. 90.1).

Progress
Treatment was commenced with rifampicin and isoniazid as combination tablets and pyrazinamide (35 mg/kg). This was given for 2 months, followed by rifampicin and isoniazid for a further 4 months. The mediastinal lymphadenopathy resolved within 3 months. The patient gained 6 kg during the 6-month treatment period. Although it was considered likely that the tuberculous infection and then disease had been acquired during his 3-year stay in Pakistan,

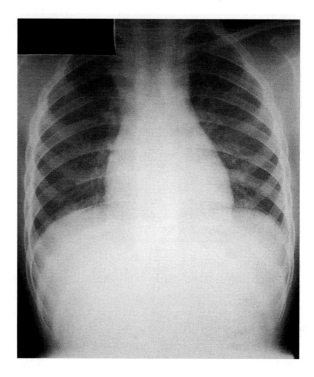

Fig. 90.1

screening of household contacts was carried out to determine whether there was a possible UK source. This revealed that the boy's 18-year-old uncle also had mediastinal lymph-node tuberculosis, and when his 84-year-old diabetic grandfather was screened shortly afterwards, he was found to have sputum-smear-positive cavitatory tuberculosis. The latter UK household case was thought to be the likely source of infection.

Comment

Primary tuberculosis is often asymptomatic in children. The degree of mediastinal lymphadenopathy can be substantial, but there may not be a visible peripheral (Ghon) focus on the X-ray. This often does not give symptoms unless there is rupture into or significant compression of a bronchus. Children are rarely infectious, but because by definition they must have been relatively recently infected, household contact tracing is appropriate in order to try to detect the source of their infection. In this case the initial assumption was that the infection had been acquired abroad, but the subsequent family screening showed a further infected adult and an infectious smear-positive adult. Other children in the family who had not lived outside the UK were also inappropriately tuberculin positive, but with normal X-rays, and were given chemoprophylaxis with rifampicin/isoniazid for 3 months.

References

American Thoracic Society. 1994: Treatment of tuberculosis and tuberculosis infection in adults and children. *American Journal of Respiratory and Critical Care Medicine* **149**, 1359–74.

Joint Tuberculosis Committee of the British Thoracic Society. 1994: Control and prevention of tuberculosis in the United Kingdom: Code of Practice 1994. *Thorax* **49**, 1193–200.

Case 91   Malaise in a 10-year-old child

Presenting complaint
A 10-year-old boy of Pakistani ethnic origin presented with a 4-week history of malaise, lethargy and evening temperature.

History of presenting complaint
The patient was born in the UK to Pakistani parents and had had a neonatal BCG vaccination. He had made a 4-month visit to Pakistan the previous year. He had been symptomatic for 4 weeks and had not responded to a course of Co-Amoxiclav. He had been screened as a household contact of a cousin with smear-positive tuberculosis 3 months earlier, when his tuberculin test (Heaf 1) was consistent with his BCG history.

Past medical history
There was no medical history of note.

Examination
The patient weighed 44.5 kg (90th centile) and his height was 156.6 cm (97th centile). There was a low-grade fever at 37.5°C and some dullness at the right base.

Tests
Haemoglobin was 12.3 g/dL, with a CRP of 71 U/L (normal range up to 6 U/L). Chest X-ray showed a right pleural effusion (Fig. 91.1) but no mediastinal glands. The tuberculin test was now much stronger (Heaf 3). Aspiration of pleural fluid was attempted but was difficult even under ultrasound control, and only 10 mL were obtained. The aspirate showed a lymphocytic exudate (protein 56 g/L) but was negative on culture. A CT scan of the thorax showed substantial pleural thickening.

Progress
Treatment with rifampicin, isoniazid and pyrazinamide as Rifater was given, with prednisolone (25 mg/day) because of the pleural thickening. The household contact was known to have fully sensitive organisms. Pyrazinamide was stopped after 2 months and rifampicin and isoniazid were given for a total of 6 months. The steroids were tailed off over 4 months. At the end of treatment there had been substantial clearance of the pleural thickening, and lung volumes were within the predicted range (FEV$_1$ 3.75/4.16; predicted value 3.15/3.43).

Comment
Pleural effusions are usually found within 6–12 months of initial infection, usually by a smear-positive adult, as is assumed in this case. In some latitudes BCG vaccination provides some protection, and it has been shown to have 65

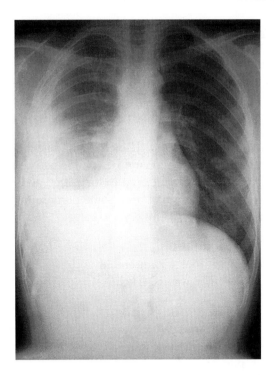

Fig. 91.1

per cent protective efficacy in children of Indian subcontinent origin born in the UK. Corticosteroids were given in addition to antituberculosis drugs because of the substantial pleural thickening. Initially it had been thought that a decortication might be needed, but this was deferred until the effects of steroids could be assessed. This child presented with non-specific general symptoms rather than specific respiratory symptoms, despite the fact that the disease was pleural.

Case 92 Partially treated bacterial meningitis?

Presenting complaint
A 21-month-old white boy was admitted with a history of 9 days of fever and vomiting.

History of presenting complaint
There was no previous medical history. The child had had a normal delivery and appropriate vaccinations (but not neonatal BCG). He had been febrile for 9 days with some vomiting. He had had amoxycillin for 7 days and erythromycin for 2 days without improvement. There had been some purposeless movements of the right arm and leg on the day of admission.

Examination
The patient was febrile at 38.2°C, miserable and pale, but showed no focal neurological signs. His weight was 10.2 kg.

Tests
Haemoglobin was 12.0 g/dL and WCC was 17.1×10^6/mL with a neutrophil leucocytosis. Chest X-ray showed some right upper zone consolidation (Fig. 92.1). Lumbar puncture showed a CSF glucose of 1.9 mmol/L (blood 4.9 mmol/L) and a WCC of 248×10^6/mL (all monocytes). Gram and ZN stains were negative, as were tests for pneumococcal and meningococcal antigens.

Progress
A diagnosis of partially treated bacterial meningitis was made, and treatment with intravenous benzylpenicillin, cefotaxime and dexamethasone (0.6 mg/kg) was started. A CT scan showed minimal dilatation of the third and lateral ventricles and no enhancement with contrast. The fever continued and a repeat lumbar puncture showed little change. A tuberculin skin test was performed and was strongly positive within 72 h. Treatment was changed to isoniazid, rifampicin and pyrazinamide, and dexamethasone was continued. A repeat CT scan now showed considerable ventricular dilatation and a ventriculoperitoneal shunt was inserted. There was a slow improvement, with one revision of the shunt being required. CSF was positive after 9 weeks on culture for M. tuberculosis, and gastric washings were negative. The organism was fully sensitive. Pyrazinamide (35 mg/kg) was given until sensitivities were confirmed. Treatment was continued with rifampicin and isoniazid for a total of 12 months. The steroids were tailed off over 3 months. The patient's weight was 13.6 kg on completion of treatment. Eighteen months after treatment had stopped he showed no neurological signs or symptoms and he started school.

Comment
Because of the rarity of tuberculous meningitis in children from low-incidence ethnic groups in low-prevalence countries, the diagnosis can be missed or

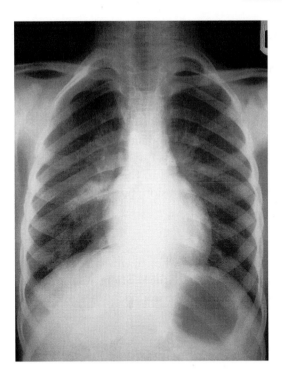

Fig. 92.1

delayed. In this case, because of previous antibiotic treatment but vomiting for 9 days, a partially treated bacterial meningitis was the initial diagnosis. Only after failure to respond to intravenous antibiotics was a tuberculin test performed, and when it was strongly positive in a non-vaccinated child the diagnosis became clear. Treatment was then given, and the early detection of hydrocephalus allowed prompt shunting, which reduces the neurological deficit. Corticosteroids were given because there had been focal signs (Stage II). Children with meningitis have invariably been infected within the previous 12 months by a sputum-smear-positive adult, often a family member. Contact tracing was immediately carried out in this family, but no household or family member source was found. The contact tracing was widened using the 'stone in the pond' principle, but despite checking over 70 adult contacts, including those with only one episode of contact, no source case was ever identified.

Reference
Palur, R., Rajshekar, V. and Chandy, M.J. 1991: Shunt surgery for hydrocephalus in tuberculous meningitis. A long-term follow-up study. *Journal of Neurosurgery* **74**, 64–9.

Case 93   A 7-year-old with cough and chest pain

Presenting complaint
A 7-year-old Pakistani girl presented with dry cough, chest pain and fever.

History of presenting complaint
The patient had had a dry non-productive cough with retrosternal pain on coughing for 4 weeks and a fever for 3 weeks. She was born in the UK and had not been abroad. An aunt who lived in the same house had just been admitted to the chest ward with a pleural effusion, possibly due to tuberculosis. There was no past history of note.

Examination
The patient was febrile at 38.1°C, her height was 115.5 cm (25th centile) and her weight 16.1 kg (below 3rd centile). There was some dullness at the right base. No BCG vaccination scar was found.

Tests
Chest X-ray showed a right pleural effusion. ESR was 70 mm/h. Mantoux 10 TU gave 20-mm induration at 72 h.

Progress
The patient was started on rifampicin and isoniazid (10 mg/kg) and pyrazinamide (35 mg/kg). The fever settled and there was X-ray resolution over the 6-month course of treatment, pyrazinamide being stopped after the first 2 months. The aunt was also found to have a tuberculous pleural effusion. Both individuals had been regular contacts of a cousin with smear-positive tuberculosis diagnosed 6 months earlier. The cousin was a daily visitor, but the household had not been given as contacts for tracing. Contact tracing revealed that this child's 8-year-old brother also had primary tuberculosis.

Comment
Virtually all children who develop a tuberculous pleural effusion have been contacts of an adult smear-positive case within the previous 12 months. Treatment with standard short-course chemotherapy is advised and pyrazinamide is safe in children and recommended by the International Union Against Tuberculosis and Lung Disease/World Health Organization (IUATLD/WHO). This case might have been preventable had the household been given as contacts. If a strongly positive tuberculin test had been found, chemoprophylaxis would have been given. Prophylaxis with either isoniazid for 6 months or rifampicin and isoniazid for 3 months is recommended for inappropriately tuberculin-positive children from high-prevalence countries found as household contacts at new-immigrant screening.

References

International Union Against Tuberculosis and Lung Disease. 1988: Anti-tuberculosis regimens of chemotherapy. Recommendations from the committee on treatment of the IUATLD. *Bulletin of the International Union Against Tuberculosis and Lung Disease* **63**, 60–4.

World Health Organization TB Unit. Division of Communicable Diseases. 1991: *Guidelines for tuberculosis treatment in adults and children in national treatment programmes*. Geneva: World Health Organization.

Case 94   Failure to thrive

Presenting complaint
An 8-year-old Asian boy was referred by the school medical service because of failure to thrive.

History of presenting complaint
The patient had been unwell for at least 6 weeks, with severe non-productive cough which was worse at night and had not responded to increased inhaler therapy. The school medical service found that his weight was 15.8 kg (less than 3rd centile) and referred him to the paediatricians.

Past medical history
The patient was born in the UK and had never been abroad. He was diagnosed as asthmatic at the age of 5 years and had had one admission at the age of 6.5 years. He was on twice-daily inhaled steroid (Fluticasone) and bronchodilator (salbutamol) by inhaler as required.

Examination
This showed the patient to be tachypnoeic with a respiratory rate of 35 breaths/min, a temperature of 38.3°C and crackles in both lungs.

Tests
Chest X-ray (Fig. 94.1) showed bilateral cavitation. Haemoglobin was 7.7 g/dL normochromic with an albumen concentration of 24 g/L. Mantoux 1:1000 was 10 mm positive. The patient was unable to produce sputum, but gastric washings were positive on microscopy for AFB and were later culture positive for M. *tuberculosis* that was fully sensitive to first-line drugs.

Progress
After the initial surprise of finding cavitatory disease in an 8-year-old, antituberculosis treatment was commenced promptly. Rifampicin and isoniazid (10 mg/kg), pyrazinamide (35 mg/kg) and ethambutol (15 mg/kg) were given. During the initial phase of treatment the patient gained 2.5 kg. Pyrazinamide and ethambutol were stopped at 2 months when the sensitivities were available. After a further 4 months of treatment with rifampicin and isoniazid a further 2.0 kg of weight had been gained, but there were some residual X-ray changes.

Comment
It is most unusual for younger children to have cavitatory, adult-type 'post-primary' disease, but the latter is seen in young teenagers, particularly from ethnic-minority groups. Standard 6-month short-course chemotherapy was given with good results, but there was some residual chest X-ray scarring, which was

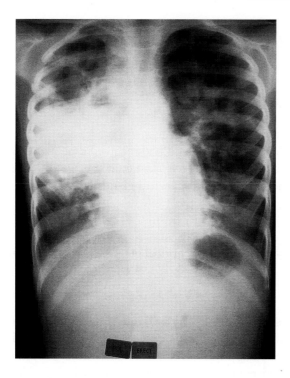

Fig. 94.1

not surprising given the extent of the initial X-ray changes. Contact tracing was initiated in order to attempt to find the source. No household contact was found to have clinical disease or to have been infected. Screening at the primary school showed no inappropriately tuberculin-positive children in the patient's year, and none of the adults (teaching or non-teaching) was a source. At the local mosque the adults who took the child's group for religious tuition were also shown not to be sources.

Case 95   Cervical lymphadenopathy

Presenting complaint
A 13-year-old Asian girl presented with a history of persistently swollen cervical glands for 3 months.

History of presenting complaint
The patient was born in the UK and had received a neonatal BCG vaccination. She had made one 6-month visit to Pakistan at the age of 10 years. She had had painless enlargement of the right cervical glands for 3 months without systemic features.

Examination
This showed non-fluctuant right cervical glands, 3 cm in diameter, in the jugular chain.

Tests
Haemoglobin was 12.3 g/dL, ESR was 4 mm/h and *Toxoplasma* antibodies were not detected. A cervical gland biopsy for histology and bacteriology was performed. The histology showed several tuberculoid granulomata, some with central necrosis and many Langhans' giant cells. Chest X-ray was normal.

Progress
The patient was started on Rifater, but 3 weeks later she developed a generalized rash. Drugs were stopped and the rash settled. At this stage the node biopsy was culture positive for M. *tuberculosis*. The rash was thought to be likely to be due to pyrazinamide, so treatment with rifampicin, isoniazid and ethambutol (15 mg/kg) was started without problems. Sensitivity results showed the organism to be highly resistant to isoniazid but sensitive to the other drugs. Isoniazid was stopped and treatment with rifampicin and ethambutol was given, supervised by the patient's parents for 12 months. Follow-up for 12 months showed no recurrence.

Comment
The surgeon who saw the child initially was more concerned that she might have had lymphoma than that she had tuberculosis, but still correctly sent half the biopsied gland for culture. Although ethnic-minority children born in developed countries have a lower incidence of tuberculosis than similar children immigrating from high-prevalence countries, their rate of tuberculosis is still substantially in excess of that found among indigenous white children. As with adults from the same ethnic groups, persistent lymphadenopathy lasting for longer than 4 weeks should still be regarded as tuberculosis until proved otherwise. Children in ethnic-minority groups have a rate of drug resistance similar to that of adults in the same ethnic group. Culture confirmation, allowing

sensitivities to be determined, is important as it both confirms the correct mycobacterial infection, excluding atypical mycobacterial infection, and allows correct drug therapy to be administered with appropriate regimens.

Cross references

Chapter 6, Section 6J, Lymph-node disease; Chapter 4, Drug resistance; Chapter 10, Environmental mycobacteria

Case 96   The infant with hyperinflation of a lung

Presenting complaint

A 9-week-old infant presented to her practitioner with a cough and shortness of breath. A diagnosis of lower respiratory tract infection was made and the child was treated with an antibiotic. She failed to improve and started to lose weight. After 1 week her mother took her back to the practitioner, who noted that the child was more tachypnoeic and that there was decreased ventilation over the left lung. The child was referred for investigation.

History of presenting complaint

The infant had been delivered by uncomplicated vertex delivery, with a birth weight of 2.9 kg, and had experienced no respiratory distress at birth. She fed normally and gained weight as expected. There was no illness in the family, and in particular the baby was not in contact with any adult with active pulmonary tuberculosis.

Examination

On examination, the length and head circumference were in the 25th percentile, with the mass on the third percentile indicating recent weight loss. The baby had a BCG vaccination scar on the upper right arm. There was no lymphadenopathy. The infant was distressed, with a respiratory rate of 70 breaths/min, and there was a chest-wall retraction. The left side of the chest was more prominent than the right side, but the excursion of the chest during breathing was greater on the right side than on the left. The trachea was deviated to the right, while on percussion the left side of the chest was hypertympanic with reduced cardiac dullness. On auscultation the air entry was normal over the right lung but was completely absent over the whole of the left lung. There was no hepatosplenomegaly.

The clinical picture was compatible with hyperinflated left chest as a result of a pneumothorax, a ball-valve obstruction of the left main bronchus, or congenital lobar emphysema.

Tests

The chest radiography (Fig. 96.1) revealed a hyperinflated left lung with a shift of the mediastinum to the right side. The radiograph was interpreted as being compatible with congenital lobar emphysema of the left lung.

The full blood count was normal for the child's age, and the arterial blood gases on breathing room air revealed a Pao_2 of 5.6 kPa and a raised $Paco_2$ of 6.5 kPa, indicating type-2 respiratory failure. The induration after the Mantoux skin test (5 IU of Japanese purified protein derivative) was 11 mm, while a barium swallow failed to indicate that there were any masses compressing both the oesophagus and the trachea.

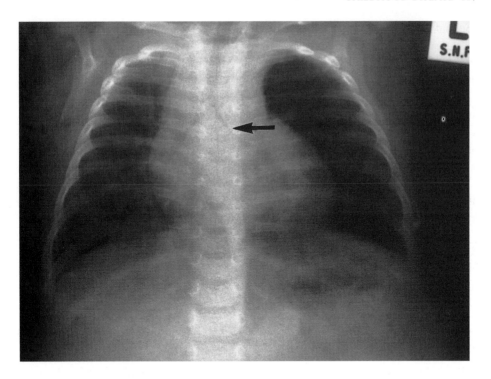

Fig. 96.1

Due to the fact that the diagnosis was uncertain, a bronchoscopy was performed which revealed that the left main bronchus was 90 per cent occluded at the level of the left upper lobe. The airway was occluded by a mass outside the bronchial wall. A biopsy was not performed but bronchial specimens were collected. A CT scan of the chest was performed which revealed hilar adenopathy compressing the airway. The radiological picture was indicative of primary tuberculosis (see Fig. 96.1). M. *tuberculosis* was cultured from the bronchial specimen, confirming the diagnosis.

Progress
The infant was treated with isoniazid (10 mg/kg/day), rifampicin (10 mg/kg/day) and pyrazinamide (20 mg/kg/day) for 6 months. Prednisolone (2 mg/kg/day) was added to this regimen for the first 3 months and then tapered. The patient responded rapidly and was discharged after 10 days. At follow-up 1 month later ventilation in the left lung was normal, and after 2 months the chest radiography showed equal aeration of both lungs. The child recovered completely.

Comment
This case highlights a number of issues concerning tuberculosis in young infants. First, large-airway compression is more common in young infants (41 per cent of cases) compared to older children (11 per cent) with pulmonary tuberculosis

(Schaaf *et al.*, 1993, 1995). On the other hand, hyperinflation of a lobe of lung as a result of hilar adenopathy causing a ball-valve effect is uncommon. In a study of 195 children with culture-proven or probable tuberculosis hyperinflation was not found in a single case (Schaaf *et al.*, 1995).

Obstruction of the large airways in small children can cause severe respiratory failure requiring ventilation and surgical decompression (Heyns *et al.*, 1998). The Mantoux skin test is of only limited diagnostic value in infants, as it has only been found to be positive in 26 per cent of infants with culture-proven tuberculosis.

Tuberculosis glandular obstruction should be considered in the differential diagnosis of infants with severe fixed airway obstruction or hyperinflation of a lobe or lung.

References
Heyns, L., Gie, R.P., Kling, S. *et al.* 1998: Management of children with tuberculosis admitted to a paediatric intensive care unit. *Paediatric Infectious Diseases* **17**, 403–7.

Schaaf, H.S., Gie, R.P., Beyers, N. *et al.* 1993: Tuberculosis in infants less than 3 months. *Archives of Disease in Childhood* **69**, 371–4.

Schaaf, H.S., Beyers, N., Gie, R.P. *et al.* 1995: Respiratory tuberculosis in childhood: the diagnostic value of clinic features and special investigations. *Paediatric Infectious Diseases* **14**, 189–95.

Editor's note
The dose of isoniazid (10mg/kg/day) is higher than that recommended in the UK.

Case 97   Chronic otorrhoea

Presenting complaint
A 15-month-old boy presented with chronic otorrhoea and a swollen neck.

History of presenting complaint
The mother brought the child for examination with complaints of fever and conjunctivitis of recent onset and chronic otorrhoea lasting for more than 4 months. This had previously been treated with antibiotics with no response. The neck became swollen and the child lost weigh (confirmed by his growth chart).

Past medical history
The patient was born at gestational age 35 weeks, with a birth weight of 2.06 Kg. The pregnancy was uneventful and the mother's serological test for syphilis was negative. The infant was breastfed, received a BCG vaccination in the neonatal period and all other immunizations were up to date. A recurrent history of diarrhoea was noted. His father had had pulmonary tuberculosis and had completed treatment 6 months previously. The patient was put on isoniazid chemoprophylaxis for tuberculosis, but treatment was not supervised.

Examination
Physical examination revealed severe bilateral otorrhoea and massive bilateral (2–3 cm, multiple) cervical lymph adenopathy, as well as inguinal and axillary adenopathy. Conjunctivitis was present and the tonsils were enlarged. A papular facial rash and severe Candida nappy rash were present. Respiratory, cardiovascular and abdominal examinations were normal. The central nervous system was intact, but developmental milestones were delayed.

Tests
Haemoglobin was 10.1 g/dL and WCC was 12.8×10^6/L with a normal differential. Total protein was 91 g/L with globulin 51 g/L. A broadened mediastinum was seen on the chest radiograph (Fig. 97.1). The lateral chest radiograph was normal, and the lateral radiograph of the neck revealed calcified lymph nodes (Fig. 97.2). The Mantoux test was performed but not read. M. tuberculosis was cultured from swabs from both ears and Staphylococcus aureus was cultured from eye swabs. Enzyme-linked immunosorbent assay (ELISA) and Western blot for HIV infection were positive. The CD4 helper-cell count was 1140/μL. The mother's HIV ELISA serology was positive.

Outcome
Treatment with isoniazid, rifampicin and pyrazinamide for 6 months was initiated, and the child was referred to the local authority health clinic. The

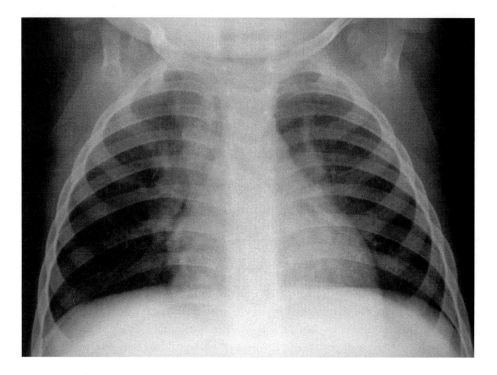

Fig. 97.1 A prominent right hilum and a broadened mediastinum suggestive of hilar and mediastinal adenopathy.

mother and child absconded, but returned to hospital 4 months later, at which stage the child had severe malnutrition, was still not walking at 19 months of age and still had bilateral otorrhoea. On clinical examination the child was found to have hepatosplenomegaly and eczematous skin lesions. A repeat chest radiograph showed enlarged hilar lymph nodes. M. *tuberculosis* sensitive to isoniazid and rifampicin was cultured from three gastric aspirates. The child was admitted to a tuberculosis hospital for 6 months for completion of anti-tuberculosis treatment. Four months after completion of therapy the family was lost to follow-up.

Comment

Like their adult counterparts, children with HIV infection are more prone to developing tubercular disease and most probably also extrapulmonary tuberculosis. This case is interesting because tuberculosis is not often considered in the differential diagnosis of chronic otorrhoea. Cervical lymph nodes in progressive primary tuberculosis tend to rupture through the skin and cause scrofuloderma, but in this patient the nodes became calcified – these could be the retropharyngeal nodes. The treatment advised for tuberculosis in children with HIV infection is the same as that for individuals without HIV infection, but

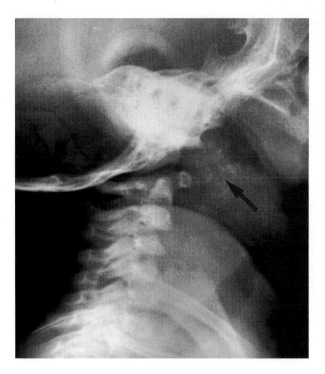

Fig. 97.2 Lateral radiograph of the neck demonstrating widened prevertebral space with calcified nodes (see arrow).

although drug resistance is not as a rule more common in HIV-infected individuals, a prolonged course of directly observed treatment (9–12 months) should be considered.

Cross reference
Chapter 8, HIV-associated disease.

HIV-associated disease

Case 98 A Romanian child

Presenting complaint
A 7-year-old Romanian child presented with weight loss, malaise, fever and cough.

History of presenting complaint
The child had failed to thrive for several months, with weight loss and poor appetite. More recently there had been mild fever and a dry cough.

Past medical history
The child was one of a twin pregnancy, and both siblings were known to be HIV positive. The other twin had died at the age of 4 years.

Examination
There was marked weight loss, the child weighing only 8 kg (predicted weight 21 kg). There was hepatosplenomegaly, generalized lymphadenopathy, some abdominal distension and delayed psychomotor development. There were scattered crackles in both lungs.

Tests
ESR was 100 mm/h, and total WBC was 8.5×10^6/mL. Chest X-ray showed nodular shadowing in all lung zones (Fig. 98.1). The tuberculin skin test was negative. Gastric washings were negative on microscopy for AFB.

Progress
Because disseminated tuberculosis was strongly suspected, quadruple therapy with daily rifampicin, isoniazid, pyrazinamide and streptomycin was given for 3 months. This was followed by rifampicin and isoniazid for a further 6 months. There was good clinical and X-ray improvement. Isoniazid was continued as secondary prophylaxis, but 6 months later fever, cough and general deterioration

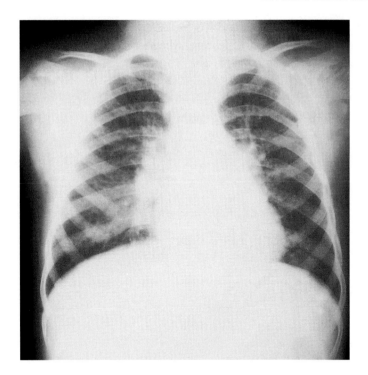

Fig. 98.1

occurred. Chest X-ray showed paratracheal lymphadenopathy. Quadruple therapy with rifampicin, isoniazid, pyrazinamide and ethambutol was given for 4 months, followed by rifampicin and isoniazid for a further 2 months with clinical improvement and radiological resolution. No anti-HIV drugs were available.

Comment

This case highlights some of the problems and also the impact of HIV infection in low-resource countries. In children who tend to have paucibacillary forms of disease even when immunocompetent, antituberculosis treatment may have to be given empirically on clinical suspicion. Because of the increased risks of both reactivation and reinfection, secondary prophylaxis with isoniazid is sometimes used. However, drug resistance is more common in HIV-positive subjects, and such single-drug prophylaxis could increase the likelihood of developing drug resistance. Trials of chemoprophylaxis are being undertaken in parts of the world where there is a high HIV/tuberculosis interaction.

References

International Union Against Tuberculosis and Lung Disease. 1991: Tuberculosis in children. Guidelines for diagnosis, prevention and treatment. A statement of the scientific committee of the IUALTD. *Bulletin of the International Union Against Tuberculosis and Lung Disease* **66**, 61–7.

Raviglione, M.C., Narain, J.P. and Kochi, A. 1992: HIV-associated tuberculosis in developing countries: clinical features, diagnosis and treatment. *Bulletin of the World Health Organization* **70**, 515–26.

Cross reference
Chapter 7, Childhood disease

Case 99 An African student

Presenting complaint
A 38-year-old student from Malawi was admitted with a history of weight loss for 1 month and more recent fever and breathlessness.

History of presenting complaint
The patient had been living in the UK for 2 months. He had lost over 6 kg in weight, and had developed fever and progressive breathlessness over a period of 4 weeks.

Previous medical history
There was a history of longstanding sensory neural deafness requiring a hearing aid.

Examination
The patient was tachypnoeic, febrile at 38.0°C and showed signs of a right pleural effusion. There was sinus tachycardia at 120 beats/min, and blood pressure was 110/80 mmHg. Jugular venous pressure was raised to 9 cm with no peripheral oedema. There was generalized lymphadenopathy and the patient's liver edge was palpable 3 cm below the costal margin. The patient weighed 45 kg.

Tests
A chest X-ray revealed miliary shadowing with some coalescence of areas into nodules. There was a right pleural effusion and a globular heart suggestive of pericardial effusion. Haemoglobin was 5.6 g/dL, the neutrophil count was 0.7×10^6/mL and the platelet count was 48×10^6/mL. Serum sodium was low at 123 mmol/L but creatinine and urea were raised at 254 μmol/L and 15.4 μmol/L, respectively. A pleural diagnostic tap showed clear yellow fluid which was positive for AFB on microscopy.

Progress
The patient was immediately started on quadruple antituberculosis chemotherapy with rifampicin, isoniazid, pyrazinamide and ethambutol with pyridoxine (10 mg) and prednisolone (40 mg) daily. He became confused and a CT brain scan and lumbar puncture were performed which were both normal. He was rehydrated and transfused with 7 units of blood. He responded well to treatment and was fit to return to the hostel in which he was living after 2 weeks of antituberculosis therapy. When he was seen at follow-up he had gained 10 kg in weight and his antituberculosis drug dosages were increased accordingly.

The patient's HIV disease was assessed. His CD4 count was 100/mL (normal range 775–1385 mL). He was therefore started on cotrimoxazole prophylaxis against *Pneumocystis carinii* pneumonia. His viral load was massively increased at 1.5 million copies/mL (log 6.4). Antiretroviral treatment would normally have been given on these values, but as he was returning to Malawi, where the drugs were either unavailable or too expensive, he decided not to start any antiretroviral therapy.

Comment

In patients with HIV disease there is often more than one obvious clinical site involved with tuberculosis. Patients may present with pulmonary and pericardial disease, as in this case, or occasionally they may present with meningeal plus pulmonary disease. Although this case was seen prior to the HIV epidemic, HIV-positive individuals appear to be more likely to develop multi-site disease, and this may reflect both the level of immune suppression and the likelihood of developing a bloodborne dissemination. Antituberculosis medication must be regularly reviewed with appropriate dosage adjustments in individuals who have gained weight. This is particularly important when patients are being given fixed-combination tablets such as Rifater or Rifinah.

There are some data to suggest that tuberculosis makes HIV disease progress more rapidly by increasing HIV viral load. This effect is probably exerted through an immunological mechanism whereby tuberculosis is producing more of the cytokine, tumour necrosis factor, which acts on a nucleo-promoter, leading to increased HIV viral replication. Controlling the tuberculosis may lead to a corresponding fall in HIV viral load independent of starting any antiretroviral therapy. After treatment this patient's viral load was 1.5 million copies/mL, putting him at great risk of developing other opportunistic infections. If he had been started on antiretroviral therapy, there would be problems with regard to drug interactions with rifampicin (see Table 99.1). Rifampicin as an enzyme inducer will affect the metabolism of many antiretroviral drugs. The important ones are the protease inhibitors, such as Saquinavir, Ritonavir, Indinavir and Nelfinavir, and the non-nucleoside reverse-transcriptase inhibitors, such as Delaviridine, Nevirapine and Efavirenz. Patients should not take rifampicin with these medications as the metabolism of these drugs will be induced and suboptimal treatment will result. Some authorities have therefore suggested that Rifabutin can be substituted for rifampicin and that Rifabutin can be used with the protease-inhibitor Indinavir, but not with Ritonavir or Saquinavir, and that it can be used with the non-nucleoside Efavirenz. Neither rifampicin nor Rifabutin shows major interactions with the nucleoside reverse-transcriptase inhibitors such as AZT, d4T, ddI and ddC.

Finally, antiretroviral therapy is not readily available in the developing world because of its cost (around $US 10 000/year for highly active antiretroviral therapy consisting of three compounds), which is obviously beyond the reach of virtually all HIV-positive patients in those countries.

Table 99.1 Central Disease Control (CDC) Guidelines for the treatment of tuberculosis in HIV-infected patients taking protease inhibitors

---

Option 1. Discontinuation of protease inhibitor for 6 months
 Discontinue the protease inhibitor
 Administer standard short-course antituberculosis treatment for 6 months
 Restart protease inhibitor after completion of antituberculosis therapy

Option 2. Discontinuation of protease inhibitor for 2 months
 (M. *tuberculosis* isolate *must* be sensitive to isoniazid and ethambutol)

 Discontinue the protease inhibitor
 Administer four-drug antituberculosis treatment for 2 months with rifampicin,
  isoniazid, pyrazinamide and either ethambutol or streptomycin
 Restart protease inhibitor
 Continue antituberculosis therapy with isoniazid (15 mg/kg) and ethambutol (50
  mg/kg) twice weekly for a further 16 months

Option 3. Coadministration of Indinavir with Rifabutin
 (cannot be recommended for patients receiving Saquinavir or Ritonavir)

 Ensure that the patient is taking Indinavir reliably (800 mg every 8 h)
 Substitute Rifabutin (150 mg/day) for rifampicin and treat tuberculosis for 9 months
  with four-drug regimen
 Monitor serum Rifabutin levels if possible

Reference
Anonymous. 1996: Clinical update. Impact of HIV protease inhibitors on the treatment of HIV-infected tuberculosis patients with rifampicin. *Morbidity and Mortality Weekly Report* **45**, 921–5.

Cross references
Chapter 6, Section 6A, Pleural effusion; Chapter 6, Section 6C, Pericardial disease; Chapter 6, Section 6G, Miliary disease

Case 100   Another fever from Africa

Presenting complaint
A 25-year-old African secretary presented with cough, malaise, fever and night sweats.

History of presenting complaint
The patient had had symptoms for 2 months. Initially she had experienced a persistent cough with white sputum associated with night sweats. She had seen two private practitioners during the first month of her illness and had received courses of amoxycillin and erythromycin. There had been a temporary improvement after erythromycin, but the symptoms had worsened in the second month, with fever, weight loss and pleuritic anterior chest pain. On direct questioning the patient complained of painful burning sensations in her feet.

Past medical history
The patient had been the main carer for her husband when he was treated for smear-positive pulmonary tuberculosis the previous year.

Examination
The patient was thin but not acutely unwell. She had oral candidiasis but no Kaposi's sarcoma. A full physical examination was unremarkable.

Tests
A chest X-ray was unremarkable. Three sputum samples were negative for AFB on ZN staining.

Progress
An HIV-related respiratory infection was suspected. A course of cotrimoxazole was prescribed and the patient was asked to consider HIV testing. After 2 weeks she had worsening symptoms and she was now pyrexial and tachycardic. There were no new signs and chest X-ray was still normal. In view of her persistent symptoms she was asked to resubmit sputum samples and antituberculosis treatment was started with the locally recommended standard modified regimen and pyridoxine. After 2 weeks the patient's respiratory symptoms were much improved and her fever had resolved. However, she complained of increasing pain in her legs which responded to treatment with amitriptyline. She accepted counselling for HIV testing, and both she and her husband were found to be HIV positive. The diagnosis of tuberculosis was confirmed 6 weeks later by positive cultures for M. tuberculosis.

Comment
Smear-negative pulmonary tuberculosis is a particularly challenging diagnostic problem in resource-poor countries where mycobacterial cultures are seldom

routinely available. In this case the cultures were performed as part of an externally funded research project. The differential diagnosis of chronic cough unresponsive to routine antibiotics in an HIV-positive patient is a broad one. It includes other opportunistic infections, such as *Pneumocystis carinii* (present in sub-Saharan Africa, but less commonly found in AIDS patients than in developed countries), cryptococcus and cytomegalovirus, and malignancies, e.g. Kaposi's sarcoma and lymphocytic interstitial pneumonitis. In addition, other causes of chronic cough should be considered, such as chronic obstructive airways disease, heart failure due to HIV-related cardiomyopathy, and post-nasal drip from chronic sinusitis. Many of these diagnoses cannot be confirmed in a setting with poor investigation facilities and non-existent microbiology and histopathology. Treatment is therefore often empirical of necessity, and locally appropriate treatment algorithms may be written to guide clinical management. Many of these algorithms include radiological criteria to support the diagnosis of smear-negative pulmonary tuberculosis. However, in the era of HIV it is now well recognized, as in this patient, that the chest X-ray of smear-negative, culture-positive tuberculosis patients may be atypical and can even be normal. With increasing immunosuppression in HIV the classical cavitating pneumonias with upper-lobe involvement are seen less commonly, with the pattern becoming more diffuse, likely to affect the lower zones and showing mediastinal lymphadenopathy. These radiographic appearances can overlap considerably with other conditions in the differential diagnosis, e.g. *Pneumocystis carinii* pneumonia (PCP) or pulmonary Kaposi's sarcoma. A history of dry cough and breathlessness may distinguish PCP clinically, and the presence of oral or cutaneous Kaposi's sarcoma increases the likelihood of pulmonary involvement with the tumour, although this can occur in isolation. In severely ill patients with an acute diffuse pneumonia that fails to respond to intravenous antibiotics, it may be necessary to treat empirically both for PCP, with high-dose cotrimoxazole, and for tuberculosis.

Painful sensory neuropathy is common in HIV patients and may be exacerbated by isoniazid. For this reason pyridoxine is often added to tuberculosis treatment regimens, but additional symptomatic treatment may be required.

Reference
Saks, A.M. and Posner, R. 1992: Tuberculosis in HIV positive patients in South Africa: a comparative radiological study with HIV negative patients. *Clinical Radiology* **46**, 387–90.

Cross reference
Chapter 1, Section 1B, Smear-negative, culture-positive disease

Case 101   General deterioration in an HIV-positive man

Presenting complaint
A 30-year-old African man with known HIV infection presented with a 4-week history of weakness, anorexia, fever and night sweats.

History of presenting complaint
The patient had been diagnosed as HIV positive 6 months previously following presentation with recurrent pneumonias and oesophageal candidiasis. He had had chronic diarrhoea which was controlled by regular codeine, but he had continued to lose weight. Fever and night sweats over the previous 4 weeks had persisted despite courses of chloramphenicol and cotrimoxazole. On direct questioning he admitted to a mild cough and intermittent abdominal discomfort.

Examination
The patient appeared wasted and frail, and needed the assistance of another person to walk. He was febrile at 38.0°C with firm bilateral symmetrical lymphadenopathy of the cervical, axillary and inguinal nodes. There was oral candidiasis but no Kaposi's sarcoma. Bibasal crackles in the chest and 3-cm splenomegaly were found.

Tests
Haemoglobin was 8.2 g/dL, MCV was 80 fL, ESR was 110 mm/h, and three malaria films were negative. Chest X-ray showed bilateral diffuse alveolar shadowing with no cardiomegaly or pleural effusions. Three sputum samples were negative for AFB on microscopy. An abdominal ultrasound scan confirmed the splenomegaly and showed marked enlargement of the para-aortic lymph nodes. Fine-needle aspiration of a cervical lymph node was positive for AFB on microscopy.

Progress
The patient was treated with the recommended local short-course regimen consisting of three times weekly rifampicin, isoniazid, pyrazinamide and ethambutol. There was marked symptomatic improvement, the patient's appetite returned and he mobilized independently. There was also radiographic improvement. However, 3 months into his tuberculosis treatment, he developed a severe headache and became confused. Lumbar puncture confirmed cryptococcal meningitis, but he deteriorated rapidly and died.

Comment
The increasing tuberculosis caseload of the dual HIV/tuberculosis epidemic in sub-Saharan Africa has been accompanied by a change in the pattern of disease, with a greater proportion of registered cases being extrapulmonary or sputum

smear negative than in the pre-HIV era. This patient showed evidence of widespread infection disseminated throughout the lungs and reticulo-endothelial system. In developed countries this pattern of disease in AIDS may suggest infection with atypical mycobacteria 'other than tuberculosis', but in Africa such infections are rare compared to M. *tuberculosis*. The broader differential diagnosis in this patient included disseminated Kaposi's sarcoma, non-Hodgkin lymphoma and fungal infections. Histological examination of lymph-node biopsy is often not available in a resource-poor setting, but fine-needle aspiration is a simple test which may show AFB in up to 85 per cent of tuberculous lymphadenitis in patients with respiratory disease, and it should be attempted wherever possible. In resource-poor countries, treatment for most other AIDS-related complications is not available, and a trial of empirical tuberculosis treatment may be worthwhile even when fine-needle aspiration is not available.

Cross references
Chapter 6, Section 6G, Miliary disease; Chapter 6, Section 6J, Lymph-node disease

Case 102   Dyspnoea and fever

Presenting complaint

A 35-year-old African man presented with a history of fever and night sweats, and more recent upper abdominal pain.

History of presenting complaint

Six weeks prior to presentation the patient developed a low-grade fever in association with night sweats. Three weeks later he noticed upper abdominal pain which became increasingly severe. Systematic enquiry revealed that he had lost weight, had become increasingly fatigued and breathless on exertion, and had experienced evening ankle oedema.

Past medical history

The patient had had several attacks of malaria, and 2 years earlier he had developed 'shingles' of the right chest.

Examination

The patient was thin and unwell with scars of herpes zoster in the right fourth and fifth thoracic dermatomes. There was symmetrical posterior cervical lymphadenopathy. The patient was febrile at 37.8°C. There was sinus tachycardia at 130 beats/min, and blood pressure was 100/70 mmHg. Jugular venous pressure (JVP) was elevated to the angle of the jaw with small 'a' and 'v' waves. The apex beat was impalpable, heart sounds were quiet and there was mild ankle oedema. The respiratory system was normal. The liver was tender and palpable 6 cm below the costal margin.

Tests

Chest X-ray showed cardiomegaly with clear lung fields, ECG showed a low-voltage pattern, and a large pericardial effusion with fibrous strands was seen on ultrasound. Pericardial aspirate was heavily blood-stained and did not show AFB on microscopy. Culture facilities were unavailable. HIV testing after counselling was refused. Urea and electrolytes were normal.

Progress

The patient was started on short-course chemotherapy with 2 months of daily supervised streptomycin, rifampicin, isoniazid and pyrazinamide followed by 6 months of daily isoniazid and ethambutol. Prednisolone (60 mg daily) was given for 4 weeks and tapered over the next 4 weeks to zero. The patient felt better within a few days of starting treatment, with resolution of fever and night sweats. Within 4 weeks the breathlessness and abdominal pain had disappeared. At the end of treatment the patient was well, with no abnormal signs on examination. The chest X-ray had returned to normal and there was no evidence of pericardial constriction on ultrasound.

Comment

Patients with pericardial effusion can present in a number of different ways, with chest pain (pericarditis), 'heart failure' (cardiac compression), shock (pericardial tamponade) and abdominal pain (hepatic congestion). A careful examination should reveal the tell-tale signs of a pericardial effusion, although sometimes the signs are subtle and can be missed. The diagnosis is confirmed by chest X-ray and ultrasound scan. In Africa the commonest cause of pericardial effusion is tuberculosis, usually due to rupture of a hilar node into the pericardial sac. The incidence of pericardial effusion has increased dramatically with the HIV epidemic, and the majority of cases in Africa are now associated with HIV co-infection. This case was thought to be HIV associated because of the previous zoster, but HIV testing was declined. Proving the diagnosis of tuberculous pericardium in resource-poor countries is usually impossible because AFB are rarely found in pericardial aspirates, and mycobacterial culture facilities are generally not available in district or even central hospitals. A careful clinical examination should be performed in order to rule out other causes, including malignancy (e.g. carcinoma of the breast) or Kaposi's sarcoma (inspection of buccal mucosa and hard palate are essential) and uraemia (asterixis, evidence of chronic pruritis). Measurement of blood urea concentration is useful, and an ultrasound scan may reveal fibrous strands in the pericardium which are strong pointers to a diagnosis of tuberculosis.

In the presence of a moderate to large pericardial effusion, pericardiocentesis should be a safe procedure in the hands of an experienced operator. However, diagnostic pericardiocentesis is rarely helpful unless mycobacterial culture facilities are available. In the presence of pericardial tamponade, or with an obviously distressed or toxic patient, pericardiocentesis should be performed to relieve pericardial compression and to exclude a pericardial empyema. In the pre-HIV era, the use of adjuvant high-dose steroid therapy was shown to decrease mortality and reduce the need for repeat pericardiocentesis, and it is now considered essential in association with short-course antituberculosis treatment. Although steroid therapy appears to be safe and beneficial in HIV-positive patients, this has not yet been confirmed in controlled clinical trials.

Cross reference

Chapter 6, Section 6C, Pericardial disease

Case 103   They thought it was *Mycobacterium avium intracellulare*

Presenting complaint
A 28-year-old white homosexual man presented with night sweats, fever and weight loss.

History of presenting complaint
The patient was known to be severely immunosuppressed with a CD4 count of less than 25/mL (normal range 775–1385/mL). He had recently been successfully treated for *Pneumocystis carinii* pneumonia, but since discharge from hospital 2 months earlier he had developed severe night sweats, fever, lethargy and malaise. He had lost 4 kg in weight and had mild diarrhoea. He had no cough or breathlessness.

Past medical history
The patient had been HIV positive for at least 10 years and was on no current antiviral treatment (previously he was taking zidovudine (AZT) and didanosine (DDI)). He had no history of tuberculosis and had had a BCG vaccination at the age of 13 years.

Examination
The patient was thin and his temperature was 39.0°C. He had widespread small lymph nodes, his spleen was palpable and he had some oral thrush, but there were no other abnormal physical signs.

Tests
The patient's chest X-ray showed paratracheal lymphadenopathy confirmed by CT scan. Haemoglobin was 9.5 g/dL with an MCV of 120 fL. WBC was 4.2×10^6/mL with a lymphocyte count of 0.3×10^6/mL. Platelets, urea and electrolytes were normal. Alkaline phosphatase activity was twice normal at 310 IU/L (normal range 50–140 IU/L). Abdominal ultrasound showed his spleen to be enlarged at 20 cm, some para-aortic lymphadenopathy and a mildly enlarged liver of homogenous texture.

Blood cultures for bacteria were negative.

Progress
Mycobacterial blood cultures were positive at 10 days. Because of the patient's severe immunosuppression and systemic features it was thought that he had disseminated *M. avium* infection, and treatment with clarithromycin and ethambutol was started. He continued to deteriorate and 1 week later

intravenous amikacin was added. Symptomatically the patient improved a little but his liver function deteriorated further, with his alkaline phosphatase activity becoming five times higher than normal and his AST activity increasing to three times its normal value.

The laboratory telephoned to say that they had cultured M. *tuberculosis* and the patient's treatment was changed to standard quadruple chemotherapy with rifampicin, isoniazid, pyrazinamide and ethambutol. His fever continued and he required transfusion for anaemia. Two weeks after the identification of M. *tuberculosis*, sensitivities became available and showed that this was a multi-drug-resistant strain. Resistance was reported to rifampicin, isoniazid, streptomycin, ciprofloxacin and ethionamide. The patient was switched to ethambutol, cycloserine, clarithromycin, pyrazinamide and clofazimine. He began to improve after 4 weeks, his fever and night sweats disappeared, and he remained well on treatment 18 months later. The laboratory informed the physicians that a case with a similar pattern of drug resistances had been reported several months earlier. The physicians discovered that these two patients had been on the ward at the same time, and restriction fragment length polymorphism (RFLP) patterns confirmed that their strains were indistinguishable from one another.

Comment

Patients with HIV infection are at increased risk of developing M. *tuberculosis*, either from reactivation or from a new infection. This patient had been exposed to someone with sputum-positive tuberculosis whilst recovering from another opportunistic infection, and had almost certainly been infected at that time. Outbreaks of MDR-TB have been reported from institutions where HIV-positive patients are looked after together. These include hospitals, clinics, prisons and shelters. HIV-positive patients who are infected with M. *tuberculosis* can progress rapidly to disease. This patient developed disseminated M. *tuberculosis* within 2 months of being exposed. The commonest cause of bacteraemic mycobacterial infection in HIV-positive patients is M. *avium*, which usually presents with sweats, fever, anaemia and hepatosplenomegaly. This usually responds within 1 month to clarithromycin and ethambutol with or without rifabutin. What is interesting is that this patient showed some response after starting amikacin to which his M. *tuberculosis* was sensitive. About 10 per cent of all patients with M. *tuberculosis* who are HIV positive will have disseminated disease with positive blood cultures. These tend to be individuals with severe immunosuppression.

If it is unsuspected or treated incorrectly, then the mortality rate of MDR-TB can be as high as 80 per cent. Risk factors for a poor prognosis from MDR-TB are low CD4 count and appropriate treatment being delayed beyond 2 weeks after the diagnosis. This patient was treated with five (reducing to three) anti-mycobacterial drugs to which the organism was sensitive. Guidelines for the treatment of drug resistance are listed in Table 103.1.

Table 103.1 Potential regimens for patients with tuberculosis with various resistance patterns

Resistance	Suggested regimen	Duration of therapy (months)*
H (+S)	R, Z, E, AMK	6–9
H and E (±S)	R, Z, AMK, OFL or CIP	6–12
H and R (±S)	Z, E, AMK, OFL or CIP	18–24
H, R and E (±S)	Z, OFL or CIP, AMK plus 2	24
H, R, Z and E (±S)	OFL or CIP, AMK plus 3	24

Key: AMK, amikacin; CIP, ciprofloxacin; E, ethambutol; H, isoniazid; OFL, ofloxacin; R, rifampicin; Z, pyrazinamide.

* These are guidelines only, and the clinical and microbiological status during treatment should be taken into consideration.

Other drugs with antituberculosis activity that are available include azithromycin, clarithromycin, ethionamide, prothionamide, clofazimine, cycloserin, capreomycin and para-aminosalicylic acid (PAS). Thiacetazone should be avoided in HIV-positive patients (fatal Stevens Johnson syndrome).

All drug treatment for MDR-TB, both as an in-patient and as an out-patient, should be fully supervised by DOT throughout.

Reference

Fischl, M.A., Daikos, G.L., Uttamchandani, R.B. et al. 1992: Clinical presentation and outcome of patients with HIV infection and tuberculosis caused by multiple-drug-resistant bacilli. *Annals of Internal Medicine* **117**, 184–90.

Cross references

Chapter 4, Drug resistance; Chapter 6, Section 6G, Miliary disease; Chapter 8, HIV-associated disease; Chapter 10, Environmental mycobacteria

Complicatioons

Case 104   Fatal consequences

Presenting complaint
A 69-year-old white man was admitted with an 18-month history of malaise, weight loss, cough and sputum production.

History of presenting complaint
The patient lived in poor social circumstances, and over the preceding 18 months had lost over 20 kg in weight, and had developed a cough with sputum but no haemoptysis. He had developed anorexia and malaise more recently over a period of 2 months. He smoked 20 cigarettes a day but did not drink alcohol.

Past medical history
There was no medical history of note.

Examination
The patient was cachectic (body weight 44 kg), wasted and toxic. There were scattered crackles in the lungs.

Tests
Chest X-ray (Fig. 104.1) showed widespread soft shadowing with cavitation. Haemoglobin was 11.5 g/dL and WBC was 5.3×10^6/mL. Serum sodium was reduced at 130 mmol/L. Three sputum samples were positive on microscopy for AFB. Blood gases on breathing air showed a P_{O_2} of 7.1 kPa and P_{CO_2} of 3.84 kPa.

Progress
The patient was immediately started on prednisolone (50 mg/day), rifampicin, isoniazid and pyrazinamide, with multi-vitamins plus pyridoxine (10 mg/day), and was given supplementary oxygen and enteral feeding. Despite these supportive measures, steroids and antituberculosis drugs, the patient died 8 days after admission. M. tuberculosis was grown from his sputum in 3 weeks, and was fully sensitive.

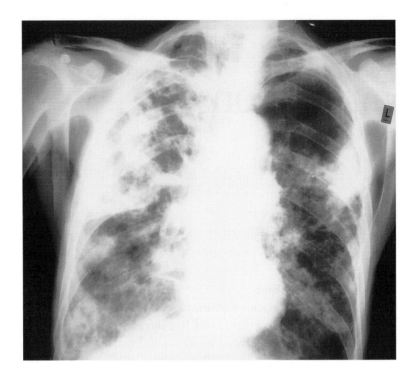

Fig. 104.1

Comment

Tuberculosis, particularly pulmonary tuberculosis, still carries a significant mortality despite the availability of adequate antituberculosis drugs. Studies have shown four separate factors to be correlated with death (by multiple regression analysis). These are increasing age, sputum-smear positivity, the number of zones involved on X-ray, and the presence of cavitation. These factors can be used to obtain some idea of the likely mortality in a given situation. This man, in whom all four adverse factors were present to a high degree (age 69 years, sputum-smear positive, 5/6 zones involved on X-ray and cavitation), had a less than 50 per cent statistical probability of survival even with prompt, full and effective treatment. Where services and medication are less efficient, e.g. in under-resourced countries, mortality may be increased by those factors as well.

References

Cullinan, P. and Meredith, S.K. 1991: Deaths in adults with notified pulmonary tuberculosis. *Thorax* **46**, 347–50.

Doherty, M.J., Spence, D.P.S. and Davies, P.D.O. 1995: Trends in tuberculosis in England and Wales; the proportion of deaths from non-respiratory disease is increasing in the elderly. *Thorax* **50**, 976–9.

Humphries, M.J., Byfield, S.P., Darbyshire, J.H. *et al.* 1984: Deaths occurring in newly notified patients with pulmonary tuberculosis in England and Wales. *British Journal of Diseases of the Chest* **78**, 149–58.

Nisar, M. and Davies, P.D.O. 1991: Trends in tuberculosis mortality. *Thorax* **46**, 438–40.

Case 105   A case of haemoptysis

Presenting complaint

A 27-year-old woman, who had been treated for tuberculosis previously, presented with a cough and haemoptysis.

History of presenting complaint

The patient was mildly mentally handicapped and had been treated for smear-positive pulmonary tuberculosis 5 years previously. The organisms had been fully sensitive, and she had been given standard short-course chemotherapy which had been supervised by her father. Treatment had been uneventful, but she had been left with some residual cavitation and scarring in the right upper lobe. For the previous 4 weeks she had had sputum and haemoptysis but no weight loss or fever.

Examination

The patient had bronchial breathing in the right upper zone.

Tests

Chest X-ray showed increased density in the right upper lobe with a halo shadow above the dense area at the site of previous cavitation (Fig. 105.1), highly suggestive of aspergilloma.

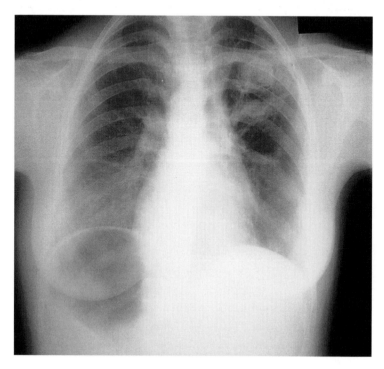

Fig. 105.1

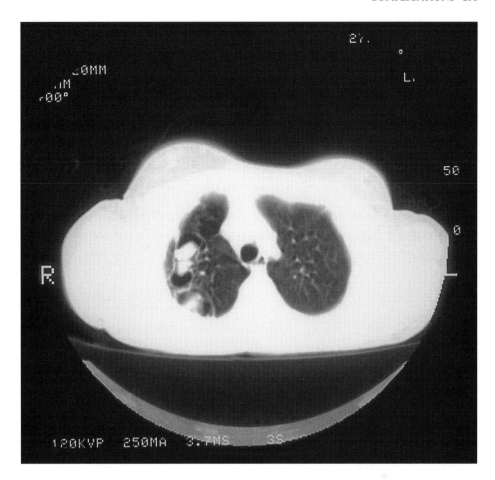

Fig. 105.2

Sputum was negative on microscopy and culture for AFB. Surprisingly, serum precipitins for *Aspergillus* were negative even on repeat testing. A CT scan of the thorax (Fig. 105.2) confirmed two separate cavities with aspergillomata.

Progress
The patient was unable to perform standard lung function tests, but was not breathless on walking for 2 km on level ground. She was referred for thoracotomy, during which dense adhesions were found between the right upper lobe and the chest wall. After these had been divided a standard right upper lobectomy was performed, and the postoperative course was uneventful. Histology confirmed aspergillomata in bronchiectatic cavities.

Comment
The development of fungal balls, usually due to *Aspergillus fumigatus* in the northern hemisphere, is a risk with lung cavitation of any aetiology, although

tuberculosis remains the commonest cause. In this case the area of cavitation was not extensive, and the patient's age and otherwise good lung function allowed a curative resection. Not infrequently in such cases, because of the degree of damage and poor lung function, surgical resection is not an option. Haemoptysis can be frequent, and is occasionally massive and fatal. Intra-cavitatory treatments with antifungal drugs are not successful. Radiotherapy of the area has been used to kill the fungal ball and fibrose vessels, and selective bronchial artery embolization has been used for treatment of haemoptysis. Secondary amyloidosis can develop with longstanding aspergillomata.

Reference
Al-Majed, S., Ashour, M., Al-Kassimi, F.A. *et al.* 1990: Management of post-tuberculous complex aspergilloma of the lung: role of surgical resection. *Thorax* **45**, 846–9.

Case 106   Persistent cough and sputum

Presenting complaint
A 57-year-old man presented with cough and haemoptysis.

History of presenting complaint
The patient had had a productive cough with > 50 mL sputum daily since the age of 19 years. He was a lifelong non-smoker. On the day of admission he had had a brisk haemoptysis of approximately 200 mL. He had not had haemoptysis previously.

Past medical history
The patient had had extensive bilateral cavitatory tuberculosis at the age of 19 years.

Examination
The patient's fingernails were clubbed with bilateral coarse crackles in the mid and lower zones. His weight was 71.5 kg.

Tests
Haemoglobin was 15.2 g/dL, and platelets and coagulation tests were normal. Chest X-ray (Fig. 106.1) showed bilateral bibasal cystic bronchiectasis with some

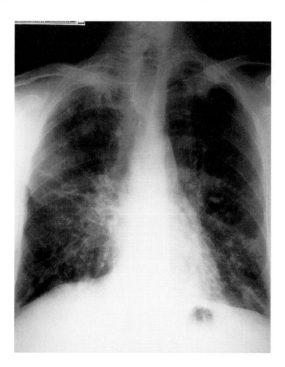

Fig. 106.1

involvement of the mid zones. Three sputum samples were negative for AFB on microscopy and subsequently on culture. *Aspergillus* precipitins were negative.

Progress

The patient was treated empirically with ampicillin and clarithromycin for 1 week, and was also given tranexamic acid for 1 week. The haemoptysis settled within 36 h and did not recur. Lung-function testing showed severe airflow obstruction (FEV_1 0.95/1.9 L, predicted value 3.64/4.61 L). The patient was given bronchodilators and inhaled corticosteroid through a high-volume spacer device.

Comment

Damage to the bronchi caused by endobronchial tuberculosis can cause airflow obstruction. The proportion of patients with airflow obstruction after treatment depends on age, sex and ethnic group. Smoking, increasing age and increasing extent of disease are all associated with airflow obstruction. The presence of one factor doubles and the presence of two factors quadruples the proportion with airflow obstruction. Chronic cough and sputum due to bronchiectatic damage (as in this case) can also accompany such airflow obstruction. Cor pulmonale can also occur as a late consequence of pulmonary damage following extensive airflow obstruction or extensive fibrosis.

Reference

Snider, G.L., Doctor, L., Demas, T.A. *et al.* 1971: Obstructive airway disease in patients with treated pulmonary tuberculosis. *American Review of Respiratory Diseases* **103**, 625–40.

Case 107   A case of tuberculosis with adult respiratory distress syndrome

Presenting complaint

A 27-year-old Thai woman presented with a 1-month history of fever and breathlessness before admission to hospital.

History of presenting complaint

Six months before her admission, the patient had been diagnosed as suffering from systemic lupus erythematosus (SLE) according to the criteria of nephritis, arthritis, malar rash plus positive ANA and anti-DNA. Following this diagnosis, she was treated with prednisolone and cyclophosphamide. The treatment continued for 5 months, after which all of the symptoms subsided and the prescription was tailed off. One month before admission, the patient developed a low-grade fever, breathlessness with dry cough and night sweats. A chest X-ray revealed miliary pulmonary infiltration bilaterally, which was predominant in both lower lobes with no cardiomegaly (Fig. 107.1).

Examination

A physical examination showed a temperature of 38.3°C, a respiration rate of 36 breaths/min and a pulse rate of 110 beats/min. The patient's general appearance

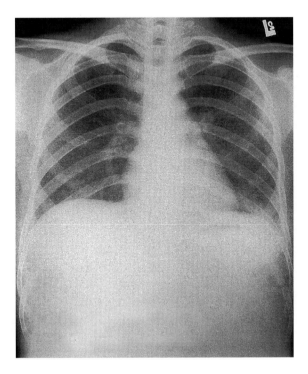

Fig. 107.1

was quite normal, except that she was rather pale. No superficial lymphadeno-pathy or oral thrush was detected, but a fine crepitation was noted in the chest on both sides. Other systems showed no abnormalities.

Tests

A chest X-ray revealed miliary infiltration on both lung fields. The complete blood count showed a haemoglobin level of 10.4 g/dL, white blood count of 7.9 × 10⁶ cells/L (4–11 × 10⁶) and a differential neutrophil count of 94 per cent.

The patient's sputum sample for AFB was positive. She was then treated with three antituberculous drugs, namely isoniazid (INH), rifampicin and pyr-azinamide. Twelve hours after treatment had started she became increasingly breathless and developed cyanosis. Arterial blood gas analysis revealed pH 7.446, Pa_{O_2} 53 mmHg, Pa_{CO_2} 31 mmHg and HCO_3 21 mmol/L even when the patient was wearing an oxygen mask with a 10-L/min bag. She was eventually intubated and placed on a respirator in the intensive care unit. Repeated chest X-rays showed progressive alveolar infiltration bilaterally (Fig. 107.2).

Outcome

The patient's haemodynamic status was kept constant with minimal fluid intake. No excessive fluid imbalance occurred during the course of her stay in hospital.

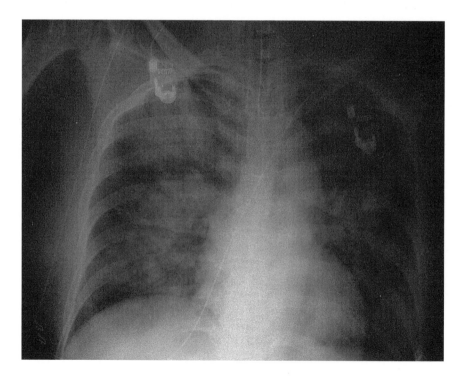

Fig. 107.2

As her bowel function was poor, and before her condition deteriorated, two second-line drugs, namely amikacin and ofloxacin, were stepped up parenterally. Neither gas exchange nor lung compliance improved despite the application of 15 cmH$_2$O of peak end expiratory pressure (PEEP) and inspired oxygen FiO$_2$ 1.0, and she died 2 weeks after admission. Prior to her death it was observed that her liver function was not in any way affected by the five drugs administered, and was normal with no sign of liver-cell damage.

Comments

The overall incidence of tuberculosis associated with adult respiratory distress syndrome (ARDS) is 1.5 to 2 per cent. Both miliary tuberculosis and tuberculosis pneumonia have been reported to cause acute respiratory failure. Most patients at high risk for developing ARDS have at least one predisposing factor, such as alcoholism, previous history of tuberculosis, postpartum, immunocompromised host, postsurgery, sarcoidosis, or either a large burden of micro-organisms or extensive pulmonary infiltration. The incidence of tuberculosis with ARDS is approximately 20 times higher in the miliary form than in tuberculosis pneumonia. The problem in distinguishing tuberculosis from other causes of ARDS, such as Gram-negative sepsis, is that there are no pathognomonic features, but fortunately we have two clinical clues for high-index suspicion of tuberculosis with ARDS, namely insidious onset of symptoms before developing ARDS, or hypotension (which is a rare occurrence in tuberculosis). The mechanism of tuberculosis-induced ARDS which is similar to Gram-negative sepsis is an immunological reaction. M. *tuberculosis* has a cell-wall component, lipo-arabinomannan, which can activate macrophage to release tumour necrosis factor (TNF)-alpha and interleukin-1-beta, in addition to making endothelial cells more susceptible to the toxic effects of TNF-alpha and also increasing intercellular adhesion molecule-1 (ICAM-1) on endothelial cells, which plays a significant role in binding neutrophils to endothelial cells.

Most first-line antituberculous drugs that are administered orally may prove ineffective in patients who suffer from gut malfunction, making it doubtful whether these patients have obtained an adequate therapeutic serum level of these antituberculous agents. In such cases, parenteral second-line antituberculous drugs such as aminoglycosides and quinolones may be added to the treatment. Nevertheless, the mortality rate of tuberculosis as the cause of ARDS is high. It is therefore extremely important, in view of the reversible nature of this disease, to give supportive treatment and chemotherapy early to reduce mortality.

References

Dyer, R.A., Chappell, W.A. and Potgieter, P.D. 1985: Acute respiratory distress syndrome associated with miliary tuberculosis. *Critical Care Medicine* **13**, 12–15.

Levy, H., Kallenbach, J.M., Feldman, C., Thornburn, J.R. and Abramowitz, J.A. 1987: Acute respiratory failure in active tuberculosis. *Critical Care Medicine* **15**, 221–5.

Environmental mycobacteria

Case 108   Cough, sputum and haemoptysis

Presenting complaint
A 62-year-old white man presented with weight loss, cough and haemoptysis.

History of presenting complaint
The patient had smoked 20 cigarettes a day since adolescence, and had had chronic obstructive pulmonary disease (COPD) for 5 years. He had experienced an increased cough for 3 months, with streak haemoptysis and weight loss of 5 kg.

Examination
A bilateral wheeze was detected with occasional crackles in the right upper zone.

Tests
Chest X-ray (Fig. 108.1) showed shadowing in the right upper zone with cavitation. Haemoglobin was 13.3 g/dL and ESR was 46 mm/h. Sputum was microscopy positive 2+ for AFB.

Progress
The patient was started on rifampicin, isoniazid, pyrazinamide and ethambutol. Sputum was culture positive for mycobacteria at 4 weeks, but there had been no significant X-ray change. At 7 weeks the identity of the organism was shown to be M. kansasii with in-vitro sensitivity to rifampicin, ethambutol, streptomycin and ethionamide, but with resistance to isoniazid. Resistance to pyrazinamide was assumed. Pyrazinamide and isoniazid were stopped and treatment was continued with rifampicin and ethambutol (15 mg/kg) for 9 months. Cultures were negative after 2 months. The cavity closed and there was only residual scarring at the right apex. FEV_1 at completion of treatment was 1.45/3.05 L. Over a 5-year period of follow-up with regular sputum monitoring there was no recurrence. The patient continued to smoke, and he died of respiratory failure due to COPD 10 years later.

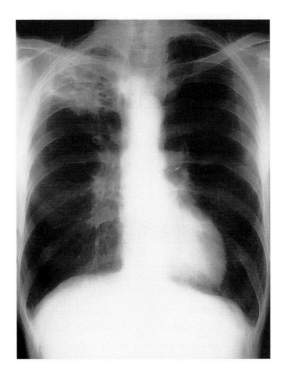

Fig. 108.1

Comment

M. *kansasii* is generally sensitive to rifampicin and ethambutol. Retrospective studies and prospective clinical trials have shown a response to 15-month and 9-month regimens of these two drugs, respectively. Among non-HIV-positive individuals, infection usually occurs in patients with coexisting lung damage from other diseases such as COPD, or even old tuberculous scarring. If environmental mycobacterial disease is suspected, ethambutol should be included in the initial regimen until identification is available. Genetic probes are now available to differentiate environmental mycobacteria from M. *tuberculosis*, and to distinguish between different environmental mycobacteria.

References

Banks, J., Hunter, A.M., Campbell, I.A. *et al.* 1983: Pulmonary infection with *Mycobacterium kansasii* in Wales 1970–79. Review of treatment and response. *Thorax* **38**, 271–5.

British Thoracic Research Committee. 1994: *Mycobacterium kansasii* pulmonary infection: a prospective study of the results of nine months of treatment with rifampicin and ethambutol. *Thorax* **49**, 442–6.

Case 109 Weight loss and cough

Presenting complaint
A 67-year-old white woman presented with weight loss and increased cough.

History of presenting complaint
The patient smoked 20 cigarettes a day, and had had increased cough with sputum for 2 months and weight loss of 4 kg. There had been no night sweats or fever.

Past medical history
The patient had been a smoker since the age of 15 years, and had had COPD for 5 years.

Examination
The patient was thin (weight 42 kg), and had an over-expanded quiet chest with no focal signs.

Tests
Chest X-ray showed bilateral upper zone shadowing with cavitation (Fig. 109.1). Haemoglobin was 12.7 g/dL and ESR was 54 mm/h. Three sputum samples were positive (3+) on microscopy for AFB. FEV_1 was 0.8/1.5 L.

Progress
The patient was started on rifampicin, isoniazid and pyrazinamide. Sputum was culture positive for mycobacteria at 5 weeks, but the chest X-ray was unchanged with no cavity reduction, and she was still heavily sputum-smear positive. M. avium intracellulare was confirmed at 8 weeks. In-vitro resistance to rifampicin, isoniazid, ethambutol and streptomycin was reported, resistance to pyrazinamide was assumed, and sensitivity to clarithromycin was reported. The in-vitro sensitivity results were ignored and treatment was switched to rifampicin (450 mg) and ethambutol (600 mg) once daily and clarithromycin (500 mg bd). Thereafter a slow improvement was observed. Cavity closure occurred over 6 months, by which time cultures had become negative. Two-monthly sputum tests remained negative and treatment was stopped after 24 months, with an FEV_1 of 0.4/1.2 L. The patient died of respiratory failure due to COPD 18 months later, with negative sputum cultures.

Comment
The first clue that this was a non-tuberculous mycobacterium was the lack of initial X-ray response. Because of this it was suspected that there was a non-tuberculous infection, but identification was necessary to confirm this. Now genetic probes are available for use on either cultures or microscopy-positive specimens. Despite the reported in-vitro resistance to many antituberculosis

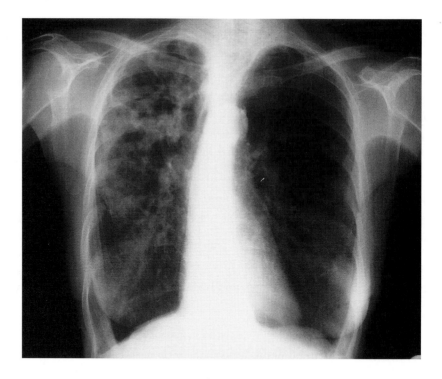

Fig. 109.1

drugs, historical controls have shown that rifampicin, isoniazid and ethambutol give a greater than 80 per cent cure rate for up to 24 months. The newer macrolides (clarithromycin and azithromycin), and the quinolone, ciprofloxacin also display action against the M. *avium* complex (and M. *malmoense*) *in vitro*. Regimens of rifampicin and ethambutol with either clarithromycin or ciprofloxacin have been successful and are currently being compared in clinical trials.

References

Hunter, A.M., Campbell, I.A. and Jenkins, P.A. 1981: Treatment of pulmonary infection caused by mycobacterium of the *Mycobacterium avium intracellulare* complex. *Thorax* **36**, 326–31.

Wallace, R.J. Jr, Brown, B.A., Griffith, A.E. *et al.* 1996: Clarithromycin regimens for pulmonary *Mycobacterium avium* complex. The first 50 patients. *American Journal of Respiratory and Critical Care Medicine* **153**, 1766–71.

Case 110   COPD with decline

Presenting complaint
A 66-year-old white man presented with malaise, cough and sputum.

History of presenting complaint
For 6 months the patient had felt less well, he had lost 5 kg in weight and he had had a poor appetite. He had experienced increased cough and sputum production but no haemoptysis. He smoked 20 cigarettes a day.

Past medical history
Three years earlier the patient had had a bleeding duodenal ulcer oversewn. An initial chest X-ray was clear, but he developed a severe left-sided postoperative pneumonia. Bronchoscopy was normal, but he was left with significant post-pneumonic scarring in the left upper zone. Cultures for mycobacteria were negative.

Examination
FEV_1 was 1.0/2.5 L. Signs of left upper zone fibrosis with tracheal deviation and crackles were found.

Tests
Chest X-ray showed left upper zone fibrosis. Sputum was sent for standard and mycobacterial cultures. One out of three cultures was positive for mycobacteria, later shown to be M. avium intracellulare with in-vitro resistance to isoniazid, rifampicin, pyrazinamide, ciprofloxacin, cycloserine and capreomycin, and susceptibility to ethambutol, clarithromycin, streptomycin and ethionamide.

Progress
Because of the lack of chest X-ray deterioration and a single culture, treatment was not started immediately. Further sputum samples were sent and two out of three cultures sent 6 weeks later were also positive. Treatment with rifampicin (600 mg), ethambutol (900 mg) and isoniazid (300 mg) was started. Cultures taken every 3 months became negative for mycobacteria. Treatment was given for 24 months. There was no X-ray change but some clinical improvement. Having had negative cultures from 3 months into treatment, those taken at cessation of treatment (after 24 months) were reported to be positive for mycobacteria (M. avium). Further cultures after another 3 months were also positive. Treatment was restarted with rifampicin (600 mg), ethambutol (900 mg) once daily and clarithromycin (500 mg bd). Cultures again became negative after 3 months, and remained negative for a further 16 months. The patient died of a myocardial infarction 19 months into his retreatment.

Comment

Most authors would recommend basing the decision to treat on more than a single culture, and usually at least two cultures separated by 2 weeks are required to confirm true infection. This man had had lung damage from a previous pneumonia which had become colonized and infected. He did well initially on rifampicin, isoniazid and ethambutol with negative cultures up to 24 months. Because of the relapse, which occurs in approximately 15 per cent of such cases with the above regimen (see Case 109), he was retreated with rifampicin, ethambutol and clarithromycin with apparent success until his death from cardiac disease. Because a high proportion of such cases are older, have lung disease and are smokers, they have a high mortality from respiratory failure and cardiovascular pathology.

Case 111 Complications of chronic lung disease

Presenting complaint
The elderly male patient was admitted with an exacerbation of COPD, and was noted to have right upper zone changes.

History of presenting complaint
The patient was a lifelong smoker with COPD. Chest X-ray had been normal in 1985, but he had been treated for presumed smear-negative tuberculosis in 1990 (see below). His chest X-ray had shown persistent shadowing in the right upper zone since that time. Because of this finding, sputum samples were sent for AFB microscopy and culture, although the patient had not lost weight or reported haemoptysis.

Previous medical history
The patient had had right upper zone X-ray changes 4 years earlier when he presented with weight loss of more than 10 kg. Bronchoscopy was negative and sputum samples were negative for AFB on microscopy, but the ESR was 126 mm/h. On antituberculosis treatment, Rifater for 2 months followed by Rifinah for 4 months, the patient gained 13 kg and his ESR fell to 25 mm/h, although cultures were negative for M. tuberculosis. There had been persistent right upper zone changes.

Examination
The patient's weight was 65 kg, he had a bilateral wheeze, and FEV_1 was 1.05/2.30 L.

Tests
One out of three of the sputum smears was positive on microscopy for AFB. Atypical infection was suspected, but no treatment was given pending cultures. All three sputum samples were culture positive for M. xenopii, which was reported with in-vitro sensitivity to streptomycin, capreomycin, ethionamide and cycloserine, borderline sensitivity to rifampicin and isoniazid, and resistance to ethambutol and pyrazinamide. Chest X-ray (Fig. 111.1) showed right upper zone scarring.

Progress
Treatment with rifampicin, isoniazid and ethambutol was started. This was given for 4 months, during which sputum cultures became negative but the patient lost 5 kg in weight. Treatment was switched to rifampicin (600 mg) and ethambutol (900 mg) once daily with clarithromycin (500 mg bd). Cultures remained negative, he regained his weight, and the X-ray remained unchanged. Treatment was stopped after a total of 24 months, with negative cultures being obtained.

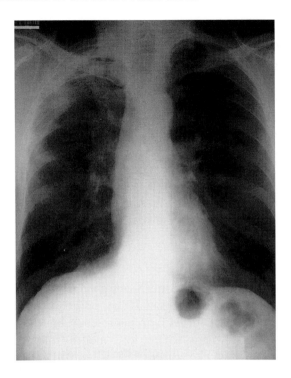

Fig. 111.1

Comment
This patient's initial illness was probably culture-negative tuberculosis, in view of the response to treatment. It is unlikely that an environmental mycobacterial infection would have responded, and so rapidly, to the combination given. Superinfection with M. *xenopii* was shown and, because of multiple positive cultures, treatment was started. Treatment regimens consisting of rifampicin, isoniazid and ethambutol have had a 70 per cent success rate, but treatment was changed to a clarithromycin-containing regimen because of the patient's continued weight loss. Clarithromycin-based regimens may be more effective, but this possibility has not been tested in clinical trials.

Reference
Smith, M.J. and Citron, K.M. 1983: Clinical review of pulmonary disease caused by *Mycobacterium xenopii*. *Thorax* **38**, 373–6.

Case 112   Discharging nodes in a child

Presenting complaint
A 4-year-old white child presented with cervical glands with discharge.

History of presenting complaint
For 2 months the patient had had a gradual increase in the right cervical tonsilar nodes which had not been altered by co-amoxiclav. These glands were multiple and one had discharged. The child was otherwise well. There was no past medical history of note, no contact with tuberculosis, and he had not had a BCG vaccination.

Examination
Right cervical nodes up to 2 cm in diameter were noted, with a small sinus.

Tests
Chest X-ray was normal, and the tuberculin test was negative. A gland biopsy was performed through the site of the sinus, with half the specimen sent for mycobacterial culture. This showed multiple discrete and confluent granulomata on histology, with scanty AFB seen. Culture grew M. *avium intracellulare* which was reported to be sensitive to clarithromycin/azithromycin but resistant to rifampicin, isoniazid, ethambutol and pyrazinamide.

Progress
This was recognized clinically as an environmental mycobacterial infection. Biopsy was performed to confirm mycobacterial histology and to obtain culture confirmation. When the erythema from the biopsy had settled 6 weeks later, an elective gland clearance was carried out, by which time culture confirmation was available. No drugs were given. The scar healed well and there were no problems and no recurrence on follow-up.

Comment
In developed countries, in children under the age of 5 years and of white ethnic origin, non-tuberculous mycobacteria are the commonest cause of discharging lymphadenopathy. Because there is a mycobacterial infection, granulomata are observed and AFB are also often seen. This can lead to confusion unless a tuberculin test is performed and some of the gland is sent for culture. The tuberculin test is usually negative or only weakly positive. Treatment with antituberculous drugs is not indicated, the appropriate treatment being excision of the affected nodes. Occasionally there is a large discharging mass, or an important structure such as the facial nerve is involved. It may then be necessary to give clarithromycin for a few weeks in order to reduce the swelling and inflammation prior to surgical clearance.

Reference
McKellar, A. 1976: Diagnosis and management of atypical mycobacterial lymphadenitis in children. *Journal of Pediatric Surgery* **11**, 85–9.

Case 113   The perils of fish

Presenting complaint
A 46-year-old man presented with skin lesions on the right antecubital fossa and hand.

History of presenting complaint
The patient had developed pinpoint lesions in his right antecubital fossa 10 weeks earlier, which had then developed over some weeks into tender raised nodules. More recently he had developed similar lesions with swelling on his right ring finger and on the dorsum of his right hand. He kept tropical fish in a 2 m × 2 m tank, and 12 weeks earlier he had cleaned out the tank and replaced the gravel.

Past medical history
Osteoarthritis was the only disorder of note.

Examination
General examination was normal. There were skin lesions in the right antecubital fossa (Plate 113.1) and similar lesions on the right ring-finger and dorsum of the hand.

Tests
One of the lesions was removed under local anaesthetic. This showed tuberculoid granulomata in the lower dermis, with Langhans' type giant cells, and scanty AFB were seen. Part of the biopsy was sent for smear and culture. An impression smear showed many AFB, and M. marinarum was later cultured.

Progress
Fish-tank granuloma was the clinical diagnosis. Once granulomata had been confirmed histologically, doxycycline treatment was commenced. However, this could not be tolerated and treatment was therefore changed to cotrimoxazole for several weeks, on which therapy the lesions resolved.

Comment
Fish-tank granulomata are seen in the developed world in individuals who keep tropical fish, but may also occur in the tropics. The organism is a fast-growing mycobacterium which responds rapidly to either doxycycline (which could not be tolerated in this case) or cotrimoxazole. There is a low recurrence rate. Reinfection can be prevented by the use of protective gloves when cleaning the tank.

Case 114   The hospital porter

Presenting complaint
A 55-year-old former hospital porter presented with pleuritic pain in the right side of his chest.

History of presenting complaint
A week previously the patient had been gardening when he noticed a sudden pain in the upper right side of his chest. He had had a cough first thing in the morning for several weeks, and had noticed that his clothes felt loose on him.

Past medical and family history
The patient's father had died of tuberculosis when the patient was 7 years old, but the patient had received no treatment for tuberculosis so far as he could remember. The patient himself smoked half an ounce of tobacco in 2 to 3 days, rolling his own cigarettes.

Examination and tests
On examination the patient was thin and had finger clubbing. There was no abnormal finding in the respiratory system. The chest X-ray showed extensive cavitation at the right apex (Fig. 114.1). Sputum was positive for AAFB on direct smear.

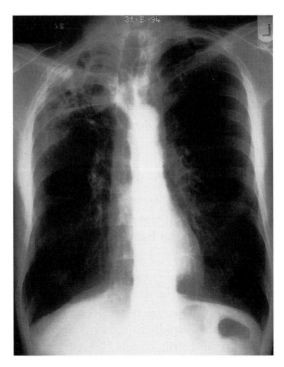

Fig. 114.1

Outcome

The patient was started on triple therapy with isoniazid, rifampicin and pyrazinamide. He was followed up monthly in the out-patient clinic and appeared to be showing some clinical improvement. Three months after presentation he was admitted with a sudden profuse haemoptysis. This settled on conservative treatment, but it was realized at the time that no culture or sensitivity confirmation had been received. A number of telephone calls were made which revealed that the local and regional laboratory had difficulty in identifying the organism. It had therefore been sent to the National Reference Laboratory, which identified the organism as M. *sulzgai*, resistant to all first-line antituberculosis chemotherapy. The patient was therefore started on rifampicin and ethambutol according to national guidelines for the treatment of environmental mycobacteria. However, after 3 months there was no clinical improvement. He continued to expectorate AAFB and to have the occasional small haemoptysis. It was therefore decided to perform a lobectomy. This was carried out with some difficulty due to the presence of extensive adhesions, and the patient was left with a fixed pneumothorax of the right apex (Fig. 114.2). In view of his lack of response to earlier chemotherapy, no antibiotics were given either during or after the operation. He remained well and the sputum was free of AAFB initially. At 3 months post-surgery sputum samples were again positive for AAFB, which were shown to be M. *sulzgai* on culture. The patient was

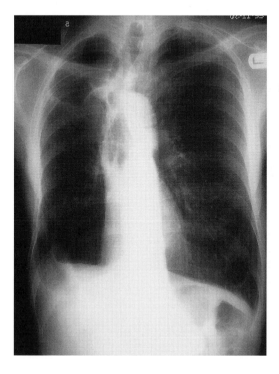

Fig. 114.2

started on a combination of rifampicin, ethambutol and clarithromycin. After 2 months his sputum became smear and culture positive. Throughout this period he remained asymptomatic and his weight remained steady. Treatment was continued for 18 months. The patient has subsequently remained free of AAFB in the sputum. He has continued his smoking habit throughout.

Comment

It is likely that this patient had had tuberculosis at some time in the past but that he had undergone a spontaneous cure. The right apex was probably cavitated, fibrotic and scarred. This presented a ready site for opportunistic infection by an environmental mycobacterium. M. *sulzgai* is a most unusual pathogen in the UK, and less than a dozen cases have been reported. It is usually quite aggressive, causing progressive lung destruction if left untreated. Like virtually all environmental mycobacteria, it was resistant to first-line therapy and probably did not respond to rifampicin and ethambutol alone. It was almost certainly a mistake not to continue some form of chemotherapy during and after surgery. It is likely that the debriding effect of surgery left 'clean lung', so that when the pathogen returned after surgery it was relatively easily eliminated by the new combination of drugs, which included clarithromycin.

Case 115   The persistent woman

Presenting complaint
A 47-year-old woman presented with haemoptysis.

History of presenting complaint
The patient had a long history of chest complaints, starting with pleurisy 20 years previously. Ten years previously she had been diagnosed as having bronchiectasis. She was otherwise well with no other relevant medical or family history. There were no abnormal physical findings and she was slightly above average weight (70 kg) for her height (165 cm).

Tests
Initial chest X-ray showed upper lobe shadowing, especially on the right, with mid zone cavitation. A CT scan confirmed widespread infiltration on the right with a 3-cm cavity (Fig. 115.1). There was also a small amount of shadowing in

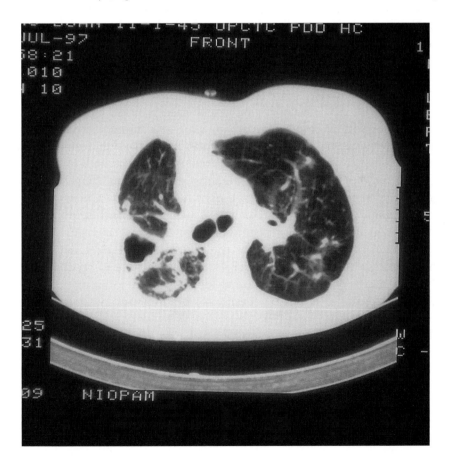

Fig. 115.1

the left upper zone. Sputum showed AAFB on direct smear. On culture, M. *avium intracellulare* was isolated. The woman had no risk factors for HIV.

Progress

The patient was initially started on triple therapy, which was changed to rifampicin and ethambutol when the organism was identified. She developed some problems with vision, so the regimen was changed to isoniazid and rifampicin. After 18 months she still felt unwell and sputum samples were persistently smear positive. All medication was then stopped for a period of 2 months. AAFB were again found in the sputum on smear and culture and M. *avium intracellulare* was isolated. The patient restarted on a regimen of ciprofloxacin and clarithromycin. Clinically she felt well on this regimen and her weight remained steady. However, over the next 12 months she had two further episodes of pleurisy and developed progressive collapse and consolidation in the right lower zone. The history of eye problems showed that no objective evidence of toxicity to the eye had been found, and rifampicin and ethambutol were added to the regimen. Four and a half years after initial presentation the patient remains clinically well and has gained a little weight (3 kg), but sputum smear and culture remain positive for M. *intracellulare*. Her chest X-ray shows progressive shrinkage of the right lung.

Comment

This patient, with previous underlying lung disease, probably bronchiectasis, has been colonized with M. *avium intracellulare* which is causing relatively asymptomatic progressive destruction of the right lung. Extensive drug regimens, which have been found to be active against M. *avium intracellulare* both *in vitro* and *in vivo*, have not been effective in eliminating the organism. Surgery has been considered to remove the cavity in the right mid zone, but in view of the fact that the patient is virtually asymptomatic it has been turned down.

This woman presents an interesting problem in management in that if the disease progresses she is likely to lose the function of the right lung. She has been on extensive medication for over 4 years. If this were to be stopped there might be a danger of spread to the other lung with further destruction. On the other hand, continued use of potentially toxic antibiotics might cause serious adverse events in time.

This case remains an intractable problem for which there appears to be no clear answer. The hope is that shrinkage and scarring in the right lung may eventually close up the cavity and lead to elimination of the organism by physical rather than pharmaceutical means.

References

Campbell, I.A. and Banks, J. 1998: Environmental mycobacteria. In Davies, P.D.O. (ed.), *Clinical tuberculosis*, 2nd edn. London: Chapman and Hall, 521–34.

Davidson, P.T. 1993: M. *avium* complex, M. *kansasii*, M. *fortuitum* and other mycobacteria causing human disease. In Reichman, L.B. and Hershfield, E.S. (eds), *Tuberculosis. A comprehensive international approach*. New York: Dekker, 505–30.

Altered diagnosis

Case 116 The cavitating judge

Presenting complaint
An 85-year-old sheepdog-trial judge presented with a sudden profuse haemoptysis.

History of presenting complaint
The patient had had tuberculosis over 40 years previously, for which he had been given a course of injections and a prolonged stay in a sanatorium. He had enjoyed good health until relatively recently, when he had begun to feel generally unwell and had lost some weight. On the day of presentation he had suddenly coughed up a large quantity of bright red blood. Initial physical examination was unremarkable.

Tests
A chest X-ray performed at presentation showed two large cavitating lesions in the right lower zone (Fig. 116.1). There was also some pleural calcification in the left upper zone. These findings were essentially confirmed on CT scan, but no new information was obtained from this investigation. Sputum was negative on direct smear for AFB. A rigid bronchoscopy showed no abnormality, and washings were negative for AAFB and cytology. Other serological tests, including ANCA, were negative.

Outcome
In view of a probable diagnosis of carcinoma and the possibility of a further profuse and potentially fatal haemoptysis, the patient was operated on and, in the absence of a clear diagnosis being available on frozen section, a right pneumonectomy was carried out. Histological examination of the specimen showed a probable diagnosis of Wegner's granulomatosis (Plate 116.1). No evidence of carcinoma or tuberculosis was found.

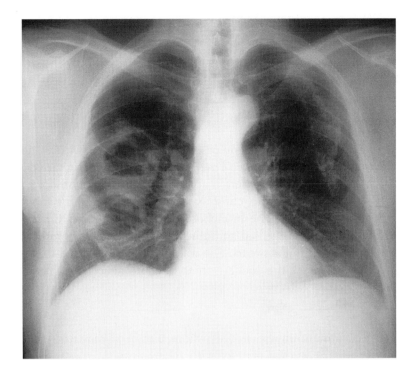

Fig. 116.1

Comment

The initial diagnosis in this patient was tuberculosis reactivation. The presence of tuberculosis in the patient's past medical history, calcification from old tuberculosis and new cavitation certainly make this diagnosis a strong possibility, although the presence of cavities in the lower part of the lower lobe makes tuberculosis slightly less likely. However, the total absence of AAFB on direct smear and bronchial washings, in the presence of extensive cavitation, makes tuberculosis extremely unlikely. When tuberculosis has caused cavitation to this extent the sputum is usually laden with bacteria.

In an elderly man who has spent much of his life with sheepdogs, hydatid cyst may be a strong possibility. The profuse haemoptysis effectively forced the surgeons to remove the whole of the right lung, as there was apparently very little useful lung tissue remaining. The diagnosis of Wegner's granulomatosis on histological examination was unexpected, especially in the presence of a negative ANCA.

Wegner's granulomatosis remains an important differential diagnosis of tuberculosis. Cavitating lesions which do not produce AAFB in the sputum should suggest the possibility of Wegner's granulomatosis. An ANCA is almost always positive and the diagnosis can usually be made by needle biopsy. The response to high-dose steroids is usually good, and excellent healing and restoration of normal lung tissue occur.

Case 117   The fertile mother

Presenting complaint
A 46-year-old mother of nine children presented with a history of 9 months of malaise and weight loss.

History of presenting complaint
The patient, who had no significant past history, presented with 9 months of progressive weight loss and malaise. Three months before presentation she had been referred to a chest clinic where a chest X-ray and bronchoscopy and CT scan had been performed. The chest X-ray had shown diffuse non-specific opacities in the right lung. The bronchoscopy and subsequent CT scan were non-contributory. The patient had continued to deteriorate with further weight loss, breathlessness and night sweats. She was eventually admitted to hospital as an emergency because of the sudden onset of more acute breathlessness and pyrexia.

Family history
The patient had nine children, two of whom had been diagnosed with cystic fibrosis. There was no known contact with tuberculosis.

Tests
The plain X-ray film taken in casualty showed diffuse shadowing throughout the right lung, particularly in the upper zone (Fig. 117.1), with a mid-zone cavity 3 cm in diameter. There was also some shadowing in the left upper zone. Sputum was initially unobtainable and the patient refused a fibre-optic bronchoscopy under local anaesthetic. Induced sputum was negative for AAFB on direct smear, and a Mantoux test (10 tuberculin units) was negative. A CT scan confirmed the presence of diffuse shadowing and a cavity in the apex of the right lower lobe. An open lung biopsy was performed. Histological examination showed a widespread inflammatory reaction, probably of infective origin. Cultures of lung tissue grew *Pseudomonas capacia*.

Comment
Because of the characteristic history and the X-ray finding, this patient was assumed to have tuberculosis. However, the absence of tubercle bacilli where a large cavity is present on chest X-ray casts considerable doubt on the diagnosis. The negative tuberculin test provided further evidence that a diagnosis of tuberculosis was probably wrong. In the absence of a firm diagnosis, and with further deterioration of the patient, a lung biopsy to obtain sufficient tissue for diagnosis was essential. Fortunately this was obtained from lung tissue culture. It is important to send biopsy specimens for culture as well as histology.

Pseudomonas capacia is a very unusual pathogen to be found in the lung of an otherwise apparently healthy adult. This patient had two children with cystic

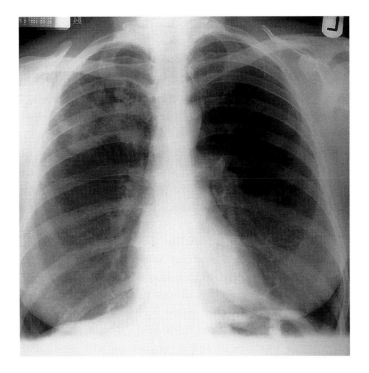

Fig. 117.1

fibrosis. She has subsequently undergone screening for cystic fibrosis but has no evidence of the disease. To detect previously undiagnosed cystic fibrosis in a 40-year-old adult would be a 'first'. No 'form fruste' of the disease or its equivalent has been described or appears to be present in this patient. It is possible that continued close proximity in caring for her children with cystic fibrosis, both of whom have *P. capacia* in their sputum, might have resulted in bacteria transferring to the mother. This in itself would be a most unusual occurrence. The organism has proved very difficult to eliminate from the mother, even with intensive antibiotic therapy. Although she has improved clinically she is still not back to normal health 18 months after the diagnosis. *P. capacia* infection remains a very uncommon differential diagnosis for tuberculosis.

Case 118   Not a tumour after all

Presenting complaint
A 65-year-old retired car worker presented with tuberculosis when the surgeon was informed by the pathologist that the lung lesion he had removed was not a tumour but tuberculosis.

History of presenting complaint
The patient had initially presented with shortness of breath and wheezing. His chest X-ray at that time was clear, and he was treated for chronic bronchitis with a combination of inhalers and antibiotics for intermittent exacerbations. He was lost to follow-up but was referred to a thoracic surgeon by his general practitioner because of increasing breathlessness. A chest X-ray taken at that time showed a 2-cm lesion in the right upper zone (Fig. 118.1). This was assumed to be a carcinoma. The patient had continued to smoke 30 cigarettes a day since his teens and throughout his illness, but because of his poor respiratory function (FEV_1 was 0.98 L, predicted value 3.15 L) the surgeon did not feel he was suitable for surgery and referred him back to his original physician for management. After 3 months of intensive out-patient treatment, including high-dose oral steroids, the patient's FEV_1 had improved to 1.65 L. A CT scan

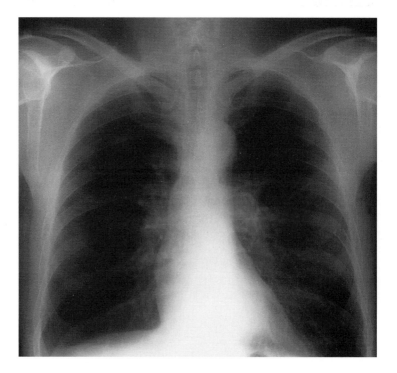

Fig. 118.1

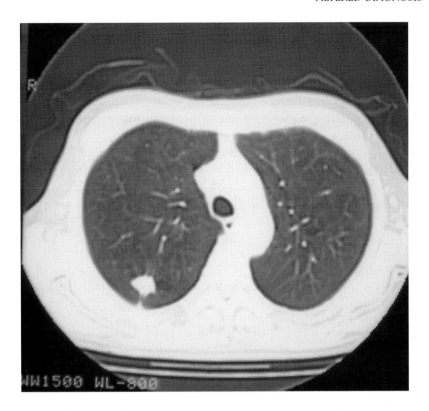

Fig. 118.2

confirmed a small lesion in the posterior segment of the right upper lobe (Fig. 118.2). A plain chest X-ray taken at the time showed no apparent change in the size of the lesion compared to 3 months earlier.

As the patient was now believed to be operable he was referred back to the surgeon and a right upper lobectomy was performed. The specimen showed histology characteristic of tuberculosis, which was positive for AAFB on staining. Sputum taken at the time of operation was also smear positive for AAFB.

Comment

Tuberculosis often mimics bronchogenic carcinoma and vice versa. There were several omissions in this patient's management, and had these aspects not been overlooked they might have prevented an unnecessary operation. At the time when this patient was referred back from the surgeon to the physician with a new lesion on his chest X-ray, a fibre-optic bronchoscopy including washings from the right upper lobe for cytology and AAFB might have provided the diagnosis.

A completely new patient presenting with such a lesion would almost certainly have been bronchoscoped before surgical referral. However, perhaps because the referral had come from a surgeon there was an implicit assumption by the physician that the patient had a carcinoma and that the role of the physician was to get the patient as well as possible for surgery, rather than to make the diagnosis.

Even sending sputum for AAFB might have provided the diagnosis, as the high-dose oral steroids might have exacerbated the tuberculosis, causing smear positivity to emerge in time.

Diagnosis of tuberculosis is often made during operation for a presumed malignancy. In a Japanese study 21 (58 per cent) of 36 patients suspected of having a malignancy had a tuberculoma at operation (Ishida et al., 1992).

A British study showed that 77 per cent of 31 patients suspected of having a malignancy in fact had tuberculosis (Whyte et al., 1989).

References

Ishida, T., Yokoyama, H., Kaneko, S. et al. 1992: Pulmonary tuberculoma and indications for surgery: radiographic and clinicopathological analysis. *Respiratory Medicine* **86**, 431–6.

Whyte, R.I., Deegan, S.P., Kaplan, D.K. et al. 1989: Recent surgical experience for pulmonary tuberculosis. *Respiratory Medicine* **83**, 357–62.

Case 119   A tuberculin-positive tumour

Presenting complaint
A 47-year-old woman presented with a 3-month history of cough, weight loss and painful joints.

History of presenting complaint
The patient had a 3-month history of cough and weight loss. During the preceding 3 weeks she had experienced painful swelling of the wrists and ankles. She smoked 40 cigarettes a day and drank half a bottle of vodka a day.

Tests
A chest X-ray (Fig. 119.1) showed a diffuse honeycomb shadow in a distinct band across the upper third of the right lung field, which on a lateral film (Fig. 119.2) and CT scan was shown to lie posteriorly. A fibre-optic bronchoscopy was entirely normal and washings were negative for AAFB and cytology. A tuberculin test (10 tuberculin units) gave 40 mm of induration.

Progress
In view of the probable diagnosis of tuberculosis, the patient was started on a triple regimen of isoniazid, rifampicin and pyrazinamide. After 2 months she was

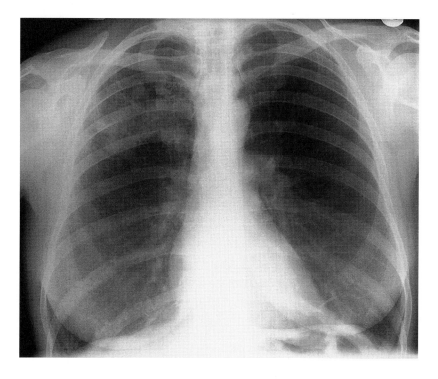

Fig. 119.1

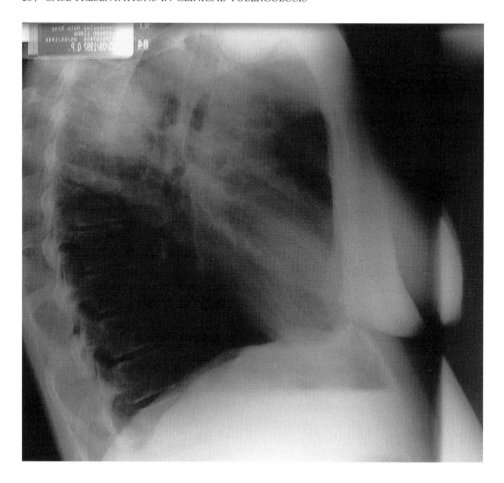

Fig. 119.2

symptomatically no better. There was slight extension of the shadowing in the right upper zone, the bronchial washings for AAFB were culture negative, and she had started to develop finger clubbing. As the diagnosis of tuberculosis was in doubt, she was referred for biopsy of the lung. This was found to be alveolar-cell carcinoma.

Comment
The very strongly positive tuberculin test result effectively caused a 2-month time loss in making the correct diagnosis, although over the long term the prognosis for alveolar-cell carcinoma is so poor that the outcome was probably not affected. It should be remembered that a positive tuberculin test is an indication of infection but not necessarily of disease. Although the degree of positivity is sometimes regarded as an indicator of active disease, there are no reliable data to support this view. It has been shown that in the elderly there is a strong correlation between pack years smoked and tuberculin positivity,

although this relationship has not been shown in individuals under 65 years of age (Nisar *et al.*, 1993).

Had the lung been biopsied transbronchially at the time of the initial bronchoscopy, the correct diagnosis would probably have been made.

Reference

Nisar, M., Williams, C.S.D., Ashby, D. and Davies, P.D.O. 1993: Tuberculin screening of residential homes for the elderly. *Thorax* **48**, 1257–60.

Case 120   A missed diagnosis

Presenting complaint
An 80-year-old man was admitted to hospital with several months' history of progressive decline, weight loss and malaise.

Progress
The patient was admitted to a general medical ward. His weight loss and malaise continued with a low-grade pyrexia. Attempts to obtain sputum were unsuccessful, and he showed no response to broad-spectrum antibiotics. His chest X-ray (Fig. 120.1) showed extensive upper zone calcification with right apical confluent shadowing and hazy shadowing in both mid zones. He progressively deteriorated and died after 10 days on the ward.

At post mortem he was found to have extensive pulmonary tuberculosis.

Comment
The chest X-ray clearly show evidence of both old and new tuberculosis. Every attempt should have been made to obtain sputum using induced sputum or tracheal aspiration if necessary. Even in the absence of confirmation, a trial of triple antituberculosis chemotherapy would have been warranted. However, if appropriate treatment had been started on admission, the outlook would still

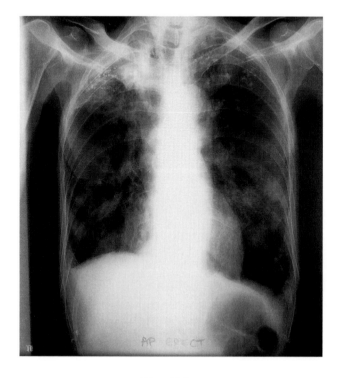

Fig. 120.1

have been poor, as tuberculosis in the frail and elderly carries a high mortality (up to 30 per cent in the over-seventies).

References

Doherty, M.J., Spence, D.P.S. and Davies, P.D.O. 1995: Trends in tuberculosis in England and Wales; the proportion of deaths from non-respiratory disease is increasing in the elderly. *Thorax* **50**, 976–9.

Humphries, M.J., Byfield, S.B., Darbyshire, J. *et al.* 1984: Deaths occurring in newly notified patients with tuberculosis. *British Journal of Diseases of the Chest* **78**, 149–58.

King, D. and Davies, P.D.O. 1992: Disseminated tuberculosis in the elderly; still a diagnosis overlooked. *Journal of the Royal Society of Medicine* **85**, 48–50.

Nisar, M. and Davies, P.D.O. 1991: Trends in tuberculosis mortality. *Thorax* **46**, 438–40.

Index